CONTENTS

*To Robert "Robby" Comfort
(one of my grandsons), who said a number of times,
"I can't wait to read this book!"*

*Special thanks to Manuel Brambila
and Stuart G. Scott.*

INTRODUCTION

The first time I visited Israel, I remember our tour guide telling us that the place we were about to visit was either a "traditional" site or an "authentic" one. Traditional meant the Jesus *may* have been there. Authentic meant that He was there for certain. For me, the difference was night and day. I was thoroughly bored with traditional sites, but *loved* standing on the shore of the Sea of Galilee and watching the sunrise, or walking through the ancient gates of Jerusalem, seeing the sites described in the Bible come to life. Years later, I still have a deep sense of joy and satisfaction that I walked in the places Jesus walked, and stood where He stood.

What I discovered in the Bible about these foods has added that same sense of joy and satisfaction to my daily meals. I *love* knowing that I'm eating what Jesus ate or recommended. And I love knowing that despite many of these foods being vilified in the past, it has come to light in recent years that every one of them is beneficial to our health. The experts had to eat their words.

I hope that you will read this publication with the same sense of discovery and excitement in which I wrote it. But keep in mind that this isn't just a book about physical food. Man doesn't live by bread alone (see Matthew 4:4). My hope is that this publication gives you food for thought about the nourishment that really matters:

> "Do not labor for the food which perishes, but for the food which endures to everlasting life…" (John 6:27)

Best wishes,
Ray Comfort

CHAPTER ONE

THE PERFECT GIFT

One of the most famous verses in the Bible predicts the virgin birth of Jesus, the promised Messiah, but the verse following it isn't so well-known:

> "Therefore the Lord himself shall give you a sign; Behold, a virgin shall conceive, and bear a son, and shall call his name Immanuel. Butter and honey shall he eat, that he may know to refuse the evil, and choose the good." (Isaiah 7:14,15, KJV)

According to this prophecy, written 800 years BC (Before Christ), Jesus would eat honey. Jesus was also given honey to eat when He appeared to His disciples after His resurrection and asked them if they had any food:

So they gave Him a piece of a broiled fish and some honeycomb. And He took it and ate in their presence. (Luke 24:42,43)

John the Baptist, the forerunner of Jesus, also ate "locusts and wild honey" (Matthew 3:4)—perhaps the honey helped to counter the taste of the crunchy insects. The Scriptures tell us that the wisest of men, King Solomon, recommended the consumption of honey to his son: "My son, eat honey because it is good, and the honeycomb which is sweet to your taste" (Proverbs 24:13).

Gratifying to the tastebuds, honey is a perfect gift to give when we want to express appreciation. Jacob told his sons to take honey with them to gain favor with a highly influential man in Egypt:

"Take some of the best fruits of the land in your vessels and carry down a present for the man—a little balm and a little honey, spices and myrrh, pistachio nuts and almonds." (Genesis 43:11)

When a queen visited the prophet Ahijah at Shiloh, she was instructed to take a jar of honey in order to gain his approval (1 Kings 14:3). Honey was also included in the gifts given to King David's army. At a time when they were hungry and weary in the wilderness, they received "wheat, barley and flour, parched grain and beans, lentils and parched seeds, honey and curds, sheep and cheese" to eat (2 Samuel 17:27–29).

Honey doesn't just leave a good taste in the mouth of those we wish to please, it is unique in that it's the only gift of food that doesn't spoil. Meat rots, bread gets moldy, fruits decompose, nuts grow stale, but honey doesn't go bad:

Natural, properly preserved honey will not expire. In fact, archeologists found honey thousands of years old in ancient Egyptian tombs, and it was still good![1]

The book of Proverbs even equates honey with healthy bones:

Pleasant words are like a honeycomb, sweetness to the soul and health to the bones. (Proverbs 16:24)

Easton's Bible Dictionary says of honey:

Canaan was a "land flowing with milk and honey" (Exodus 3:8). Milk and honey were among the chief dainties in the earlier ages, as they are now among the Bedawin; and butter and honey are also mentioned among articles of food (Isaiah 7:15). The ancients used honey instead of sugar (Psalms 119:103; Proverbs 24:13); but when taken in great quantities it caused nausea, a fact referred to in Proverbs 25:16, 17 to inculcate moderation in pleasures.[2]

The metaphor of a "land flowing with milk and honey" is used over twenty times in the Bible to

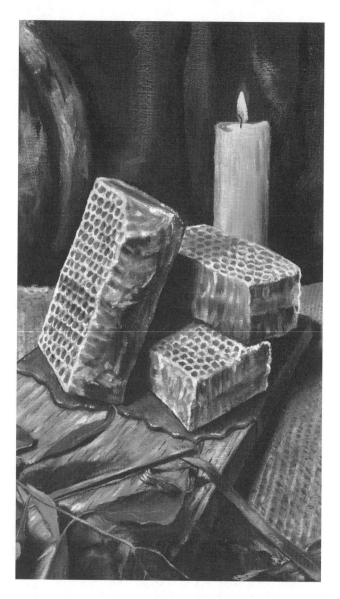

describe abundance. The book of Job uses a similar phrase, describing rivers "flowing with honey and cream" (Job 20:17).

In the book of Ezekiel, the Scriptures liken the Word of God to the sweetness of honey:

> And He said to me, "Son of man, feed your belly, and fill your stomach with this scroll that I give you." So I ate, and it was in my mouth like honey in sweetness. (Ezekiel 3:3)

Health Benefits of Raw Honey

- Dioscorides, an ancient Greek physician, wrote about honey's healing properties. He recognized that it can heal burns and spots on the face, as well as inflammation in the throat and tonsils. Honey has proven to be a more effective cough treatment than some cough medications.

- It's also a great source of energy with only 17 grams of carbohydrates in one teaspoon. It acts as an energy booster since its glucose and fructose enter directly into the bloodstream. Additionally, honey aids athletic performance because it maintains blood sugar levels that help muscle recuperation after workouts.

- Honey is a great allergy reliever. Small amounts of pollen, which is used to produce it, trigger the immune system to produce antibodies to pollen, decreasing allergic reactions.

- Honey is a great natural antiseptic, because it slowly releases hydrogen peroxide, an antibacterial, antimicrobial, and antiseptic compound that can kill germs, disinfect a wound, and heal broken skin. Honey applied to a wound keeps it moist and acts as a protective barrier against infection, making it very effective in treating cuts, burns, bug bites, yeast infections, eczema, acne, dandruff, and fungal infections.

- It helps to eliminate free radicals and toxins from the body, boosting the immune system. Free radicals are molecules that the body produces when it breaks down food or encounters pollutants. These can damage the body's cells and contribute to disease.

- It can help with weight management and loss when consumed in moderation with lemon and/or cinnamon because it contributes to the digestion of stored fat in the body. Honey's glycemic index (a measure that determines how fast food raises sugar levels) is 54–59, whereas other sugar forms can reach as high as 105.

- Honey is full of antioxidants, including organic acids and phenolic compounds, which help to stabilize free radicals.

- Honey helped lower LDL (bad cholesterol) and raised HDL (good cholesterol) during an eight-week clinical trial on diabetic patients. Furthermore, a 2013 study showed that consuming honey daily for twelve weeks improved the metabolism in type 1 diabetes patients.

- It promotes heart health because of its positive effects in lowering blood pressure, cholesterol, and triglyceride levels.

- It releases serotonin in the body, which is a neurotransmitter that improves mood and happiness. The body then converts the serotonin into melatonin, known as the sleep hormone, that regulates the sleep-wake cycle, controlling the length and quality of sleep.

- Honey, particularly tualang honey, proved in a 2015 review of studies that it improves learning and memory processes. It enhances brain areas related to memory, decreases oxidative stress in the brain, and increases brain growth factors.

- It has also proven to be helpful to boost the short-term memory of post-menopausal women. A 2011 study showed that after four months of daily taking 20 grams of honey, these women had better short-term memory than those who took hormone pills to fight a hormone-related intellectual decline.

- The Mayo Clinic affirms, "Studies suggest that honey might offer antidepressant, anticonvulsant and anti-anxiety benefits. In some studies, honey has been shown to help prevent memory disorders."

Sources:

academia.edu/3228620/Improvement_in_immedi-ate_memory_after_16_weeks_of_tualang_honey_Agro_Mas_supplement_in_healthy_postmenopausal_women

healthfitnessrevolution.com/top-10-health-benefits-honey/

ncbi.nlm.nih.gov/pmc/articles/PMC5635760/

tailormadehealth.com/organic-honey-benefits/

mayoclinic.org/drugs-supplements-honey/art-20363819

TASTEFUL QUOTE
"If you want to gather honey, don't kick over the beehive." —Dale Carnegie

CHAPTER TWO

SIX DANGEROUS SIDE EFFECTS

As we have seen in the previous chapter, the Bible tells us that Jesus ate butter along with honey:

> "Butter and honey shall he eat, that he may know to refuse the evil, and choose the good." (Isaiah 7:15)

But how could Jesus have eaten something that experts have found to be a major cause of heart disease? Surely as God in human form (see 1 Timothy 3:13), Jesus knew that butter is damaging to human health. An article titled "6 Dangerous Side Effects of Eating Too Much Butter, According to Experts" warns:

> "Butter is high in saturated fat. A tablespoon has about seven grams, which is about one-third of your daily recommended allowance," explains Leann Poston MD, MBA, MEd.

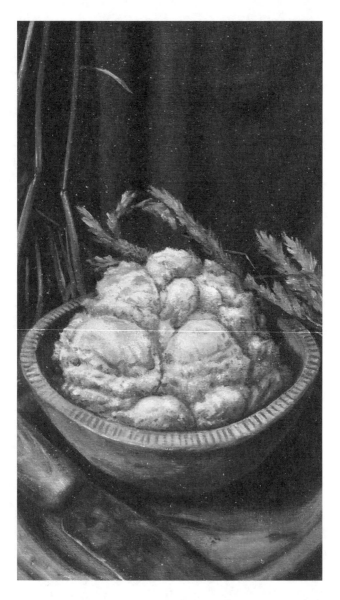

"Eating a diet high in saturated fats increases your LDL ('bad') and HDL cholesterol. Increased LDL cholesterol can contribute to atherosclerosis and atherosclerosis can increase your risk for blood clots, strokes, and heart attacks."[3]

However, in another article titled "Is Butter a Healthy Fat?" *Scientific American* has some good news for butter lovers:

Johanna writes: "I was recently surprised to hear a nutritionist encourage people to use butter, calling it a healthy fat. I've always avoided butter because of the saturated fat. Yet, a quick online search shows multiple articles saying butter is making a comeback as a healthy fat. Can this be true?"

It's true that butter contains saturated fat. It's also true that saturated fat's reputation as an artery clogger has been undergoing some rehabilitation in recent years. Diets that are high in saturated fat can raise your cholesterol levels. But...the links between saturated fat, cholesterol, and heart disease are a lot more complex than we once thought. In fact, having some saturated fat in your diet may actually be good for your heart and other organs.[4]

The *Harvard Public Health Magazine* reported similar good news. Based on findings in the *Annals of Internal Medicine*, "eating less saturated fat, the dietary demon that makes buttery croissants so irresistible, doesn't actually lower a person's risk for heart disease." The Harvard article continues:

> The finding was reported widely in the media, hitting all the cultural hot buttons: food and fat, death and disease, bacon and Brie. As Mark Bittman's column in *The New York Times* rhapsodized: "Butter is Back. Julia Child, goddess of fat, is beaming somewhere."[5]

I Can't Believe It's Not Better

When butter got a bad battering, the good news about a lookalike called "margarine" spread like wildfire. But hold your horses. The lookalike may be an imposter. Check this heart-stopping information:

> Don't let that heart-healthy checkmark on the packaging fool you—not only is margarine no better for you than butter, it may actually be increasing your risk of cardiovascular disease.[6]

> The truth is, there never was any good evidence that using margarine instead of butter cut the chances of having a heart attack or developing heart disease. Making the switch was a well-intentioned guess, given that margarine had less saturated fat than butter, but it overlooked the dangers of trans fats.[7]

Butter was labeled a bad food choice in the past because of its high saturated fat content. Various health experts started promoting margarine instead. Back in the day, margarine used to be high in trans fats. These days, it has fewer trans fats than before, but it's still loaded with refined vegetable oils.

Not surprisingly, the Framingham Heart Study showed that people who replace butter with margarine are actually more likely to die from heart disease.[8]

Health Benefits of Butter

Authors Sally Fallon and Mary G. Enig, PhD, explain the benefits of this creamy spread in "Why Butter Is Better":

Heart disease was rare in America at the turn of the century. Between 1920 and 1960, the incidence of heart disease rose precipitously to become America's number one killer. During the same period butter consumption plummeted from eighteen pounds per person per year to four. It doesn't take a Ph.D. in statistics to conclude that butter is not a cause. Actually butter contains many nutrients that protect us from heart disease. First among these is vitamin A which is needed for the health of the thyroid and adrenal glands, both of which play a role in maintaining the proper functioning of the heart and cardiovascular system. Abnormalities of the heart and larger blood vessels occur in babies born to vitamin A deficient mothers. Butter is America's best and most easily absorbed source of vitamin A.

Butter contains lecithin, a substance that assists in the proper assimilation and metabolism of cholesterol and other fat constituents.

Butter also contains a number of anti-oxidants that protect against the kind of free radical damage that weakens the arteries. Vitamin A and vitamin E found in butter both play a strong anti-oxidant role. Butter is a very rich source of selenium, a vital anti-oxidant—containing more per gram than herring or wheat germ.

Butter is also a good dietary source [of] cholesterol. What?? Cholesterol an anti-oxidant?? Yes indeed, cholesterol is a potent anti-oxidant that is flooded into the blood when we take in too many harmful free-radicals—usually from damaged and rancid fats in margarine and highly processed vegetable oils. A Medical Research Council survey showed that men eating butter ran half the risk of developing heart disease as those using margarine.[9]

Butter has other health benefits as well:

- It can help lower your chances of cancer. Butter is high in beta-carotene, a compound that your body converts into vitamin A. Beta-carotene is what gives butter its yellow color and has been linked to lowered risks of lung cancer and prostate cancer.

- It is an excellent source of nutrients such as fat, vitamin A, vitamin E, vitamin B-12, vitamin K, vitamin B2, phosphorus, and calcium.

- Butter is a powerful antioxidant because of its high levels of carotene. About 60% of carotene intake is transformed into disease-fighting compounds, providing a boost to the immune system. Carotene is also transformed in vitamin A which is fat-soluble, helping the parts of the body with membranes such as the eyes, skin, mouth, and the urinary and digestive tracts. Vitamin A promotes cell growth and reparation, and encourages the production of lymphocytes—the defensive cells that fight against viruses and autoimmune diseases.

- The high levels of vitamin A and carotene have been proven to work as anti-cancer agents. They work together against cancerous growth and promote spontaneous cell death (apoptosis) in tumors. The coagulated linoleic acid (CLA) is found in significant levels in butter, reducing the chances of getting cancer.

- Butter's good amount of beta carotene helps to protect the eyes, slow the development of cataracts, reduce the risk of macular degeneration, and decrease other eye conditions as well as angina pectoris.

- It contains high levels of glycospingolipids that protect the intestines and increase the defenses in the stomach.

- Butter and other high-fat dairy products cannot be linked with cardiovascular diseases. In fact, research has shown that high-fat dairy products can be beneficial for cardiovascular health. The National Library of Medicine states, "Despite the contribution of dairy products to the saturated fatty acid composition of the diet, and given the diversity of dairy foods of widely differing composition, there is no clear evidence that dairy food consumption is consistently associated with a higher risk of CVD."

- Butter's vitamin A is essential in the development and growth of children. A lack of vitamin A during gestation can lead to narrow faces and skeletal structure, crowded teeth, and small palates.

- Butter has more vitamin A than any other type of vitamin, which is important for a healthy thyroid. Hypothyroidism and other thyroid diseases are linked to a lack of vitamin A, causing an imbalance in the rest of the endocrine system.

- Butter's high cholesterol helps the brain and nervous system to develop properly, especially in growing children. The brain produces its own cholesterol but also pulls it from the blood's plasma which comes from the diet.

- Butter and cream carry a unique hormone-like substance called Wulzen Factor, which helps to prevent the calcification of the joints that leads to arthritis. It also protects from hardened arteries and the calcification of the pineal gland. However, the pasteurization of milk, cream, and butter removes the Wulzen Factor. It is interesting that baby calves that are given a substitute without the Wulzen Factor do not survive.

- It is rich in essential minerals, like manganese, zinc, copper, and selenium. These elements are very important to the bones' health, supporting bone repair and growth. Arthritis and osteoporosis can be prevented with a healthy butter intake.

Sources:

webmd.com/diet/health-benefits-butter#1
healthbenefitstimes.com/butter/
pubmed.ncbi.nlm.nih.gov/19259609/
dairy.com.au/products/butter

How Butter Is Made

Most of the butter we eat is made from cow's milk, and occasionally goat's milk, but that's not the case throughout the world. In other countries butter can also be made from the milk of sheep, camels, reindeer, water buffalo, llamas, yaks, and even horses.

Many of us as children gave butter making a try in a school class, learning about how the pioneers lived. Churning cream or whole milk in a wooden butter churn is a good way to develop patience, and muscles.

According to Britannica.com,

> Butter making was developed centuries ago. Ancient Sanskrit writings and the oldest books of the Bible mention the use of butter. Butter once was used as a cosmetic and tonic for the hair and skin. The Greeks and Romans used it as a medicine.
>
> Primitive churns were made of hollow logs or leather bags that were swung from trees to create churning action. Butter was also made by beating milk in a bowl. Later churns were made of jars with wooden dashers.
>
> In the United States butter making was primarily a household activity until the late 1800s. After the development of cream separators, creameries began to appear. Creameries performed the butter-making labor on the farm and stimulated greater demand for butter in the cities. With modern production

methods and transportation, butter can be shipped thousands of miles and can be stored for months without losing its flavor and quality.[10]

> **TASTEFUL QUOTE**
> *"If you're afraid of butter, use cream."*
> —Julia Child

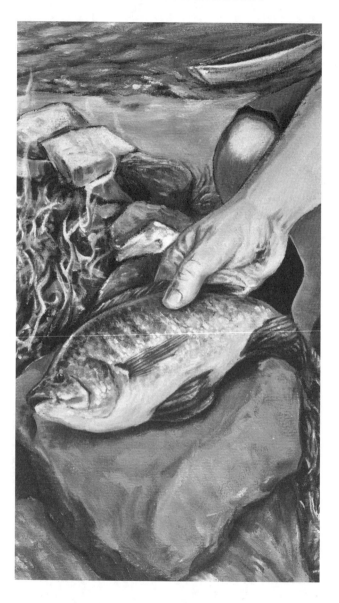

CHAPTER THREE

RESURRECTION FOOD

After Jesus died on the cross and then rose from the dead, much to the joy of His disciples, He appeared to them and asked a question: "Have you any food here?" While they were still marveling, they "gave Him a piece of a broiled fish and some honeycomb. And He took it and ate in their presence" (Luke 24:41–43).

Jesus not only ate fish, He cooked it for His disciples:

> Then, as soon as they had come to land, they saw a fire of coals there, and fish laid on it, and bread. Jesus said to them, "Bring some of the fish which you have just caught." (John 21:9,10)

There are some who find that very hard to swallow, as in this article from PETA:

If you're a Christian who follows a vegetarian or vegan diet, you may have heard this defensive response from fellow meat-eating believers: "But Jesus wasn't a vegan. He ate fish!" Although there are stories throughout the Bible that appear to suggest that Jesus ate fish, there has been serious theological debate as to whether he actually did or if the word "fish" is a mistranslation.[11]

If the word "fish" is a mistranslation, then the preceding verse in the same passage of Scripture needs to be changed. It says,

And He said to them, "Cast the net on the right side of the boat, and you will find some." So they cast, and now they were not able to draw it in because of the multitude of fish. (John 21:6)

Jesus told these fishermen to cast their fishing nets on the right side of their boat—because they had fished all night and hadn't caught any fish. If it was a mistranslation, when they pulled their net in it must have been filled to overflowing with something else. What was the mysterious something else? Fortunately, thanks to another vegan site, we're not left floundering: "the Greek word translated 'fish' may actually refer to dried seaweed as some scholars believe…"[12]

So that we can see the context of this incident, here it is directly from the Bible (*New King James Version*):

Simon Peter said to them, "I am going fishing."

They said to him, "We are going with you also." They went out and immediately got into the boat, and that night they caught nothing. But when the morning had now come, Jesus stood on the shore; yet the disciples did not know that it was Jesus. Then Jesus said to them, "Children, have you any food?"

They answered Him, "No." And He said to them, "Cast the net on the right side of the boat, and you will find some." So they cast, and now they were not able to draw it in because of the multitude of fish.

Therefore that disciple whom Jesus loved said to Peter, "It is the Lord!" Now when Simon Peter heard that it was the Lord, he put on his outer garment (for he had removed it), and plunged into the sea. But the other disciples came in the little boat (for they were not far from land, but about two hundred cubits), dragging the net with fish. Then, as soon as they had come to land, they saw a fire of coals there, and fish laid on it, and bread. Jesus said to them, "Bring some of the fish which you have just caught."

Simon Peter went up and dragged the net to land, full of large fish, one hundred and fifty-three; and although there were so many, the net was not broken. Jesus said to them, "Come and eat breakfast." Yet none of the disciples dared ask Him, "Who are You?"—knowing that it was the Lord. Jesus then came and took the bread and gave it to them, and likewise the fish. (John 21:3–13)

Here now is my own paraphrase of John 21:3–13 from *The New Vegan Version**:

Peter was going fishing, and so the disciples followed him. They fished all night and caught nothing. In the morning Jesus stood on the shore and asked if they caught any-thing. When they said that they hadn't caught any fish, He told them, "Cast the net on the right side of the boat, and you will find some." They did what He had told them to do, and were not able to pull the net in because of the amount of dried seaweed that came up from the wet ocean. The miraculous catch confirmed to Peter that it was the Lord, and so he dived into the sea to go to Jesus. The other disciples followed him in the boat, and then dragged the net filled with the dried seaweed.

But Jesus didn't apologize for it being seaweed rather than the fish He'd promised.

---

* There is no such thing as *The New Vegan Version* of the Bible. This is purely satire.

Instead, He gave them dried seaweed to eat for breakfast that He'd already been cooking on the fire. Jesus then told them to bring in the remaining seaweed, and Peter dragged it closer. It contained one hundred and fifty-three large pieces.

For those who are interested in reality, the Greek word used in this passage to describe the catch is transliterated *opsarion*, and is translated "fish."[13]

Feeding the Multitudes

Jesus also miraculously multiplied fish on two different occasions to feed hungry crowds (Matthew 14:14–21 and 15:32–38).

> Now Jesus called His disciples to Himself and said, "I have compassion on the multitude, because they have now continued with Me three days and have nothing to eat. And I do not want to send them away hungry, lest they faint on the way."
>
> Then His disciples said to Him, "Where could we get enough bread in the wilderness to fill such a great multitude?"
>
> Jesus said to them, "How many loaves do you have?"
>
> And they said, "Seven, and a few little fish."
>
> So He commanded the multitude to sit down on the ground. And He took the seven loaves and the fish and gave thanks, broke

them and gave them to His disciples; and the disciples gave to the multitude. So they all ate and were filled, and they took up seven large baskets full of the fragments that were left. Now those who ate were four thousand men, besides women and children. (Matthew 15:32–38)

On the other occasion He fed five thousand men, plus women and children. He could have miraculously created any food to give to the famished multitude, but along with bread He provided fish, a healthy protein to satisfy their hunger and nourish their bodies.

Fish in Bible Times

The Israelites ate a variety of fresh and saltwater fish, according to both archaeological and textual evidence. Remains of freshwater fish from the Yarkon and Jordan rivers and the Sea of Galilee have been found in excavations…Fishermen supplied fish to inland communities, as remains of fish, including bones and scales, have been discovered at many inland sites. To preserve them for transport, the fish were first smoked or dried and salted.[14]

Health Benefits of Fish

- Fish is one of the healthiest foods in the world, with its many important nutrients, high-quality proteins, iodine and other minerals and vitamins. It is an excellent source of omega-3 fatty acids, which are very important for our brains and reduce inflammation.

- It is a great source of protein without the high saturated fat is found in other types of meat.

- Fatty fish, such as salmon, trout, sardines, tuna, and mackerel, are considered to be the healthiest because of their omega-3 and vitamin D content. Most people lack these nutrients, which are known to prevent many diseases.

- It reduces the risk of heart attacks and strokes, the two most common causes of premature death. Studies have shown that people who consume fish regularly have a lower risk of heart attacks, strokes, and heart diseases in general. The American Heart Association recommends two servings of fish per week.

- Fish helps in reducing the bad cholesterol level in the body, according to the Baylor University Medical Center Proceedings.

- According to a review published by the *American Journal of Cardiology*, "The results indicate that fish consumption is associated with a significantly lower risk of fatal and total coronary heart disease (CHD). These findings suggest that fish consumption may be an important component of lifestyle modification for the prevention of CHD."

- Omega-3 is essential for growth and development. It is recommended that pregnant and breastfeeding women include 340 grams of salmon, sardines, or trout (low-mercury fish) per week as a source of omega-3, which is very important for the brain and eye development.

- Fish can help in delaying the normal mental decline that comes with aging, as well as prevent serious neurodegenerative conditions like Alzheimer's disease. Those who eat fish weekly have more gray matter, which is the brain's major functional tissue responsible for memory and regulating emotions.

- Fish has proved to help in preventing low mood, decreased energy, and depression. Omega-3 helps to fight depression, mental conditions, and bipolar disorder, and enhances the effectiveness of antidepressant medications.

- Fatty fish like salmon and herring are a great source of vitamin D, which is lacking in over 40% of Americans. A single serving (113 grams) of cooked salmon contains 100% of recommended daily intake of vitamin D. A tablespoon of fish oil, such as cod liver oil, provides 200% of the recommended daily vitamin D.

- Vitamin D deficiency is linked to sleep disorders. A study among 95 middle-aged men showed that consuming salmon three times a week improved sleep and daily functioning.

- Fish reduces the risk of type 1 diabetes in children and of autoimmune disease in adults, because of its omega-3 fatty acids. In children, fish also reduces the risk of asthma by 24%.

- Regular fish consumption is linked to a 42% lower risk of age-related macular degeneration (AMD) that causes vision impairment and blindness. Another study showed 53% decreased risk of wet AMD, thanks to the omega-3 found in fatty fish.

- The American College of Rheumatology has found that regular consumption of fish reduces rheumatoid arthritis.

Sources:

healthline.com/nutrition/11-health-benefits-of-fish
pubmed.ncbi.nlm.nih.gov/15110203/
ncbi.nlm.nih.gov/pmc/articles/PMC1312230/#sec1_6title
pubmed.ncbi.nlm.nih.gov/23112118/

TASTEFUL QUOTE

"Fishing is much more than fish. It is the great occasion when we may return to the fine simplicity of our forefathers." —Herbert Hoover

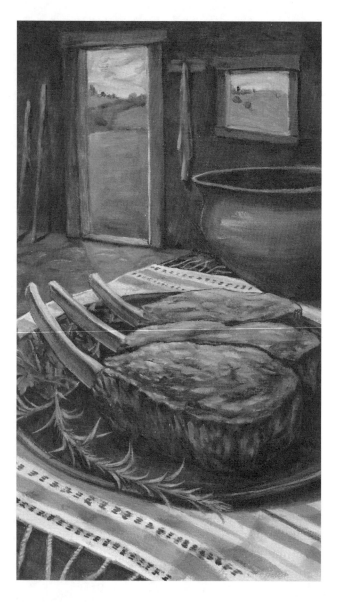

CHAPTER FOUR

ANOTHER VEGAN NIGHTMARE

Vegans will be horrified to know Jesus not only ate fish, He also ate meat. One obvious example is the Passover meal He shared with His disciples. Those who celebrated the Passover had a choice of sacrificing a lamb or young goat. Exodus 12:5 says, "Your lamb shall be without blemish, a male of the first year. You may take it from the sheep or from the goats." How then do we know that it was a lamb that was prepared for the Passover by the disciples, and not a goat? The Gospel of Mark gives us details:

> Now on the first day of Unleavened Bread, *when they killed the Passover lamb*, His disciples said to Him, "Where do You want us to go and prepare, that You may eat the Passover?"
>
> And He sent out two of His disciples and said to them, "Go into the city, and a man

will meet you carrying a pitcher of water; follow him. Wherever he goes in, say to the master of the house, 'The Teacher says, "Where is the guest room in which I may eat the Passover with My disciples?" ' Then he will show you a large upper room, furnished and prepared; there make ready for us."

So His disciples went out, and came into the city, and found it just as He had said to them; and they prepared the Passover. (Mark 14:12–16)

Perhaps it was only the disciples who ate the lamb. But Jesus Himself puts that thought to rest:

Then came the Day of Unleavened Bread, when the Passover must be killed. And He sent Peter and John, saying, "Go and prepare the Passover for us, that we may eat." (Luke 22:7,8)

Jesus didn't say that the Passover lamb was to be killed and eaten only by His disciples. He said, "…that *we* may eat."

When He told Peter and John to prepare it, they would have done so according to the clear instructions given in Scripture. The Passover was instituted by God Himself when the Israelites were dwelling in Egypt, and He specified how this special lamb was to be selected:

"Speak to all the congregation of Israel, saying: 'On the tenth of this month every man shall take for himself a lamb, according to the house of his father, a lamb for a household. And if the household is too small for the lamb, let him and his neighbor next to his house take it according to the number of the persons; according to each man's need you shall make your count for the lamb. Your lamb shall be without blemish, a male of the first year. You may take it from the sheep or from the goats. Now you shall keep it until the fourteenth day of the same month. Then the whole assembly of the congregation of Israel shall kill it at twilight." (Exodus 12:3–6)

In addition to the lamb, the disciples had to handle preparations for the rest of the meal. Experts have surmised as to what other foods would have been on the table at the Passover meal:

Scripture provides us with another clue: unleavened bread and wine were also on the menu. Jesus broke bread and blessed wine, telling his Apostles that the bread was his body and the wine was his blood—thus laying the basis for the communion.

According to Urciuoli and Berogno, other food on the table would have included cholent, a stewed dish of beans cooked very low and slow, olives with hyssop, a herb with a mint-like taste, bitter herbs with pistachios and a date charoset, a chunky fruit and nut paste.

"Bitter herbs and charoset are typical of Passover, cholent is eaten during festivities, while hyssop was also consumed on a daily basis," Urciuoli said.[15]

Preparing Lamb in Bible Times

In addition to its selection, God gave very precise instructions on how the Passover lamb was to be prepared:

> Then they shall eat the flesh on that night; roasted in fire, with unleavened bread and with bitter herbs they shall eat it. Do not eat it raw, nor boiled at all with water, but roasted in fire—its head with its legs and its entrails. You shall let none of it remain until morning, and what remains of it until morning you shall burn with fire. And thus you shall eat it: with a belt on your waist, your sandals on your feet, and your staff in your hand. So you shall eat it in haste. It is the LORD's Passover. (Exodus 12:8–11)

After the Exodus, the Israelites would observe Passover by taking the family's lamb to the temple starting at around 3 o'clock. The lamb would be properly slaughtered and its blood poured at the base of the altar by the priest. The father would then "place it over his shoulder, and carry it to the place where the family would share the meal together. There, the lamb would be roasted outside over an open fire until it was ready to eat."[16]

The Significance of the Lamb

Far more than just a meal, the sacrificial lamb was symbolic of the Messiah. Its innocence is epitomized in Jesus of Nazareth. He is called the "Lamb of God" many times in the Bible, being first foreshadowed in the book of Genesis when Abraham offered "his only begotten son" (see Hebrews 11:17):

> But Isaac spoke to Abraham his father and said, "My father!"
> And he said, "Here I am, my son."
> Then he said, "Look, the fire and the wood, but where is the lamb for a burnt offering?"
> And Abraham said, "My son, God will provide for Himself the lamb for a burnt offering." (Genesis 22:7,8)

John the Baptist recognized Jesus, the promised Messiah, as the "Lamb of God":

> The next day John saw Jesus coming toward him, and said, "Behold! The Lamb of God who takes away the sin of the world!" (John 1:29)

The prophet Isaiah, in 800 BC, spoke of Jesus and likened Him to a lamb for the slaughter:

> He was oppressed and He was afflicted,
> Yet He opened not His mouth;
> He was led as a lamb to the slaughter,
> And as a sheep before its shearers is silent,
> So He opened not His mouth. (Isaiah 53:7)

Philip the Evangelist explained Isaiah 53—about Jesus being the sacrificial Lamb—to the Ethiopian eunuch:

> Now the passage of the Scripture that he was reading was this:
>
> "Like a sheep he was led to the slaughter
>   and like a lamb before its shearer is silent,
>   so he opens not his mouth.
> In his humiliation justice was denied him.
>   Who can describe his generation?
> For his life is taken away from the earth."
>
> And the eunuch said to Philip, "About whom, I ask you, does the prophet say this, about himself or about someone else?" Then Philip opened his mouth, and beginning with this Scripture he told him the good news about Jesus. (Acts 8:32–35, ESV)

The apostle Paul said of Jesus, "For indeed Christ, our Passover, was sacrificed for us" (1 Corinthians 5:7).

On the first Passover, God instructed the Israelites to take some of the blood of the lamb and place it on the two doorposts and on the lintel of the houses where they eat it.

> "For I will pass through the land of Egypt on that night, and will strike all the firstborn in the land of Egypt, both man and beast; and against all the gods of Egypt I will execute

judgment: I am the LORD. Now the blood shall be a sign for you on the houses where you are. And when I see the blood, I will pass over you; and the plague shall not be on you to destroy you when I strike the land of Egypt." (Exodus 12:12,13)

It is the blood of Jesus, the Lamb of God, that shelters us from death so that it passes over those who trust Him:

…knowing that you were not redeemed with corruptible things, like silver or gold, from your aimless conduct received by tradition from your fathers, but with the precious blood of Christ, as of a lamb without blemish and without spot. (1 Peter 1:18,19)

Over two dozen times in the book of Revelation Jesus is referred to as "the Lamb" Here are just a few:

Then I looked, and I heard the voice of many angels around the throne, the living creatures, and the elders; and the number of them was ten thousand times ten thousand, and thousands of thousands, saying with a loud voice:

"Worthy is the Lamb who was slain
To receive power and riches and wisdom,
And strength and honor and glory and blessing!" (Revelation 5:11,12)

After these things I looked, and behold, a great multitude which no one could number,…standing before the throne and before the Lamb, clothed with white robes, with palm branches in their hands, and crying out with a loud voice, saying, "Salvation belongs to our God who sits on the throne, and to the Lamb!" (Revelation 7:9,10)

…for the Lamb who is in the midst of the throne will shepherd them and lead them to living fountains of waters. And God will wipe away every tear from their eyes. (Revelation 7:17)

And they overcame him by the blood of the Lamb and by the word of their testimony, and they did not love their lives to the death. (Revelation 12:11)

All who dwell on the earth will worship him, whose names have not been written in the Book of Life of the Lamb slain from the foundation of the world. (Revelation 13:8)

Health Benefits of Lamb

- Lamb is primarily composed of protein—about 25%. It contains the 9 essential amino acids that the human body needs for growth and maintenance.

- Lamb fat, or tallow, can contain higher levels of saturated fat than beef and pork. Saturated fat used to be considered a risk factor for heart disease, but studies have not found any relationship between them. The National Library of Medicine published an article that affirms, "A meta-analysis…showed that there is no significant evidence for concluding that dietary saturated fat is associated with an increased risk of Coronary Heart Disease or Cardiovascular Disease."

- Lamb tallow contains "ruminant trans fats," which (unlike those in processed foods) are believed to be good for the health. The most common ruminant trans fat is conjugated linoleic acid (CLA) in higher amounts than beef and veal. CLA is known for its many health benefits like the reduction of body fat mass.

- Lamb is high in calories and saturated fats, but there is evidence that eating lamb occasionally actually promotes metabolic activity and weight loss.

- Lamb contains a noteworthy quantity of omega-3 fatty acids that work as anti-inflammatories.

- Lamb meat is a great source for zinc, phosphorous, selenium, and other minerals that are necessary for bone mineral density.

- Lamb contains a variety of vitamins and minerals that are very important for numerous bodily functions. Lamb is therefore an excellent component in a healthy diet. A single serving of lamb provides about 30% of the recommended daily zinc intake—and without enough zinc, the immune system is compromised.

- *The American Journal of Clinical Nutrition* in 2000 revealed that 38% of the population suffers of a vitamin B12 deficiency. Lamb provides about half of the recommended daily B12 intake.

- It is a rich source of folic acid, which is very important for the development of babies, preventing neural defects in newborns.

- Lamb contains high amounts of beta-alanine, which is an amino acid the body uses to produce carnosine. Carnosine is a necessary substance for muscle function and has been associated with decreased fatigue and improved exercise performance. Vegetarian and vegan diets that are low in beta-alanine decrease carnosine in the muscles.

- Lamb prevents anemia because it is a great source of calcium and iron. It promotes the growth and maintenance of muscle mass, improving their function and exercise performance.

Sources:
healthline.com/nutrition/foods/lamb#nutrition
pubmed.ncbi.nlm.nih.gov/20071648/
organicfacts.net/lamb-meat.html
academic.oup.com/ajcn/article/71/2/514/4729184
#111374654

TASTEFUL QUOTE
*"Nothing is better for a man than that he should eat
and drink, and that his soul should enjoy good in his
labor. This also, I saw, was from the hand of God."*
—King Solomon (Ecclesiastes 2:24)

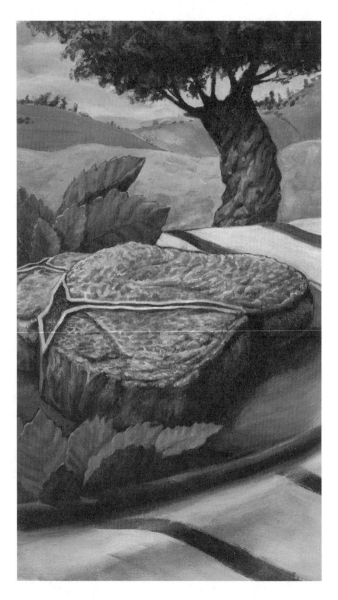

CHAPTER FIVE

FOOD OF THE HIGHEST ORDER

When Jesus told the story of "The Prodigal Son," He told us precisely how the prodigal's father celebrated:

> "The father said to his servants, '…And bring the fatted calf here and kill it, and let us eat and be merry; for this my son was dead and is alive again; he was lost and is found.' And they began to be merry." (Luke 15:22–24)

The extent to which the father was joyful is seen in his killing of the "fatted calf." His was a celebration of the highest order, and Jesus therefore had him ordering the best food he could find: veal, the tender meat from a calf. That in itself is a commendation of Jesus for veal. This wasn't mere prime rib or moist beef brisket. This was arguably the best meat human beings can eat (as we will see below under "Health Benefits"). The website "All My

Chefs," which hosts secrets of the world's best chefs, confirms veal's appeal:

> The ancient Romans were very fond of veal. It is still a popular meat in Italy today and is actually more widely consumed than beef. For a long time, eating veal was a sign of wealth: you had to be rich to afford to slaughter an animal with so little meat on it. It was also reserved for celebrations, inspired by the parable in the Bible, in which the prodigal son returns and the father kills a fatted calf in his honor.[17]

Two thousand years after Jesus told this story, we still refer to "killing the fatted calf" as a *special* celebration, "a joyful occasion or a warm welcome." The phrase even made it into a popular song, "Bennie & The Jets," where Elton John wrote, "We'll kill the fatted calf tonight so stick around."

Jesus often referred to Abraham in Scripture. Perhaps when He spoke of the joyful father celebrating by killing the fatted calf, He had a similar celebration in mind. A "tender and good" calf was killed when the Lord appeared to Abraham in Genesis 18:

> And Abraham ran to the herd, took a tender and good calf, gave it to a young man, and he hastened to prepare it. So he took butter and milk and the calf which he had prepared, and set it before them; and he stood by them under the tree as they ate. (Genesis 18:7,8)

However, this meal was much more than a typical celebration, as verse 1 tells us that "the LORD appeared to him." One of Abraham's three guests was God Almighty taking on the appearance of a man. This is known as a Christophany, a pre-incarnate appearance of Christ.

If this visitation with Abraham was indeed a Christophany, Jesus was not simply recommending the consumption of veal in the parable of the Prodigal Son, but He had eaten it Himself when it was prepared by Abraham.

Health Benefits of Veal

In the article titled, "Seven Secret Health Benefits of Veal," we are told that both beef and veal are filled with common nutrients, essential minerals and vitamins, but that veal has something unique that makes it a very healthy food.

- Veal is lower in fat than beef, and is very low in saturated fat, which we're advised to eat in limited quantities.

- Veal offers slightly more protein than beef, so for meat eaters looking for more protein, veal gets a thumbs up. Veal is also low calorie, with only 179 calories in a 3 ounce top round cut.

- Veal is enriched with B vitamins, including B-12, thiamine, riboflavin, niacin, and pantothenic acid. People who consume beef on a regular basis can easily switch to a smarter and healthy choice with veal.

- Veal can supply 2 percent of daily required sodium value with a 3-ounce top round cut, slightly more than in beef. The amount of iron is about the same.

- Like beef, veal is an excellent source of zinc, providing 25% of the zinc needed in our daily diet.

- Because it is so tender, veal is easier for our bodies to digest than beef. People who have difficulty digesting other red meats can give veal a try.[18]

Meat Preparation in Bible Times

Meat was prepared in several different ways. The most common was to cook it with water as a broth or a stew (for example, Ezekiel 24:4,5). Meat stewed with onions, garlic, and leeks and flavored with cumin and coriander is described on ancient Babylonian cuneiform tablets, and it is most likely that it was prepared similarly in ancient Israel. Stewed meat was considered to be a dish worthy of serving to honored guests (Judges 6:19,20).

A less common way to prepare meat was to roast it over an open fire, but this was done particularly for the meat of the Passover lamb. For long-term storage, meat was smoked, dried, or salted.

TASTEFUL QUOTE

"Better is a dinner of herbs where love is, than a fatted calf with hatred." —Proverbs 15:17

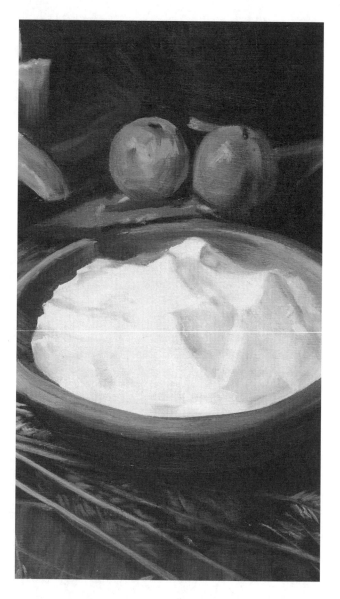

CHAPTER SIX

THE VILIFICATION OF SALT

In the Sermon on the Mount, Jesus had the audacity to say, "Salt is good" (Mark 9:50). Audacity, because there is a mountain of scientific data saying that salt *isn't* good. We are told that it is bad for human consumption, and it has been passionately vilified for the last fifty-plus years. That passion will continue as long as there are articles like this one:

> This week, 3 studies involving hundreds of thousands of patients were published in the prestigious *British Medical Journal*. All 3 studies showed the same thing, our excessive salt intake is making us sick and killing us early.
>
> A recent study by [a] Harvard Professor …concluded that 2.3 million deaths worldwide could be prevented each year if we simply reduced our salt intake.[19]

The article writer argues that too much salt in the diet is a major cause of high blood pressure, which can lead to heart attacks, strokes, dementia, blindness, kidney failure, and numerous other health problems. It can also trigger an inflammatory reaction throughout the body, increasing the risk of autoimmune diseases such as multiple sclerosis or arthritis.

However, there is some good news for those who appreciate good taste:

> Controversy over the amount of salt started approximately in 1972 when Lewis Dahl, MD, showed evidence that a diet high in sodium contributes to high blood pressure. A recent *Cochrane Collaboration* found no evidence to suggest that salt reduction did the trial participants any good or any harm…A recent study published in the *American Journal of Hypertension*, in a population-based cohort study of 8670 French adults, showed that salt consumption was not associated with elevations in systolic blood pressure (SBP), independent of gender and other multiple adjustments.[20]

> New research shows that for the vast majority of individuals, sodium consumption does not increase health risks except for those who eat more than five grams a day, the equivalent of 2.5 teaspoons of salt. Fewer than five

percent of individuals in developed countries exceed that level.

The large, international study also shows that even for those individuals there is good news. Any health risk of sodium intake is virtually eliminated if people improve their diet quality by adding fruits, vegetables, dairy foods, potatoes, and other potassium rich foods.[21]

So, it seems science is confirming that salt, in moderation, is indeed "good." In the book of Job, Job asks the rhetorical question:

"Can flavorless food be eaten without salt? Or is there any taste in the white of an egg?" (Job 6:6)

In the Sermon on the Mount, Jesus even likened His disciples to salt:

"You are the salt of the earth; but if the salt loses its flavor, how shall it be seasoned? It is then good for nothing but to be thrown out and trampled underfoot by men." (Matthew 5:13)

Calling someone the "salt of the earth" is an expression still in use today, as is saying someone is "worth their salt"—speaking of their great value. The Bible also uses salt as a metaphor for tasteful speech:

> Let your speech always be with grace, sea-
> soned with salt, that you may know how you
> ought to answer each one. (Colossians 4:6)

What Is Salt?

Salt was created by God primarily for seasoning—
for enhancing the flavor of food. Without salt, food
is bland. And so is life. Salt is good. Every salt shaker
worth its salt should carry a label that says "Recommended by the Maker."

The type of salt we consume is sodium chloride.
As a seasoning, salt has been used for at least 5,000
years, placing it among the oldest and most common seasonings. God designed our tastebuds to
detect five basic tastes, including saltiness, as well as
sweetness, sourness, bitterness, and umami (savory).

If salt were bad, why would God see fit to sur-
round our precious eyes with salt? Our tears contain
salt, as WebMD explains:

> Tears are salty because they are made from
> water from our body that contains electro-
> lytes (salt ions). Tears are 98% water. The
> remaining 2%, which is responsible for the
> salty taste, contain:
>> Oils
>> Salt
>> More than 1,500 proteins
>
> Tears and all of our other body fluids are
> salty because of electrolytes, also known as
> salt ions. Our bodies use electrolytes to create

electricity that helps power our brains and move our muscles.[22]

Salt in Bible Times

The most common and important seasoning was salt (Job 6:6), demonstrated by how it is referenced throughout the Bible, and by how its use was mandated with most sacrifices (Leviticus 2:13). Salt was obtained from the Mediterranean or the Dead Sea. It was produced by evaporating seawater from both natural and artificially created drying pans along the Mediterranean coast. It was also obtained by mining salt deposits, such as at Sodom near the Dead Sea.[23]

Health Benefits of Salt

- Salt is often enhanced with the mineral iodine, which is often removed during the purification process. Iodine plays an important role in metabolism, as it's needed for the thyroid gland. These salts are labeled "iodized" and in moderate quantities will keep the thyroid functioning properly.

- Salt helps the body to maintain good hydration levels and electrolyte balance. The muscles, tissues, and cells need water to function properly, and salt helps the body to retain the right amounts and avoid muscle cramps, dizziness, and fatigue. According to Harvard's School of

Health, "The human body requires a small amount of sodium to conduct nerve impulses, contract and relax muscles, and maintain the proper balance of water and minerals."

- Salt is used in hospitals to restore optimum hydration levels to patients who receive saline intravenously.

- The sodium in salt is important to prevent low blood pressure (hypotension), which causes nausea, dizziness, fainting, and blurry vision.

- Salt can help prevent type 2 diabetes because it strengthens the body's sensitivity to insulin that is required to maintain a fit body. Salt increases the body's ability to metabolize glucose and provide energy to the liver, muscles, and nervous system.

- It also ensures a healthy pregnancy. It should be part of a healthy diet that ensures the development of the baby.

- Salt combats sun strokes. When exposed to high heat or direct sun for a long time, the body can fail to release sufficient heat. The body temperature becomes too high causing excessive sweating in an effort to cool itself down. In the process, essential salt and water are lost through the sweat glands. Elderly people and infants are at greater risk of heatstroke and should keep their body well hydrated and consuming adequate salt to maintain their electrolyte balance.

Sources:

everydayhealth.com/diet-nutrition/diet/salt-health-benefits-risks-types-how-cut-back-more/
mayoclinic.org/healthy-lifestyle/nutrition-and-healthy-eating/in-depth/sodium/art-20045479
organicfacts.net/health-benefits/other/health-bene-fits-of-salt.html
hsph.harvard.edu/nutritionsource/salt-and-sodium/

TASTEFUL QUOTE
"One thing I like about Argentina, they only cook with salt; that's it." —Robert Duvall

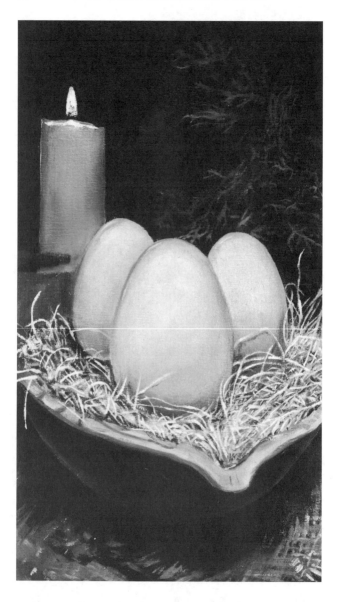

CHAPTER SEVEN

GOOD GIFTS

Jesus also had the effrontery to say that eggs were a good food to give to children. Once again you would think that He had access to the explosive amount of scientific evidence proving that eggs are a hand-grenade with the pin pulled out. One study showed:

> Eating just three to four eggs per week was associated with 6 percent higher risk of cardiovascular disease and 8 percent higher risk of any cause of death. And if you eat two eggs per day, you'd be boosting your risk of cardiovascular disease by 27 percent, and your risk of early death by 34 percent, according to the study.[24]

However, the same article said,

> The debate over eggs originated because of yolks' high cholesterol content, and previous recommendations cautioned people to eat

less cholesterol as a way to prevent cardiovascular disease, according to Alyssa Pike, R.D., manager of nutrition communications at the International Food Information Council.

However, she told *Runner's World*, daily cholesterol limits were removed from the U.S. government's 2015 Dietary Guidelines for America.

"This change came about because the current body of research about dietary cholesterol does not support the idea that dietary sources of cholesterol have a large impact on our blood cholesterol levels," she said.

Stuart Phillips, Ph.D, the director of the McMaster Centre for Nutrition, Exercise, and Health Research, agrees that the cholesterol-from-food link may not be as damning as we once thought.

"Cholesterol may be something to pay attention to, but its relationship to heart disease and death isn't huge, and there are lots of other contributors," he said. "Even the paper itself shows that it isn't really the problem."[25]

Here is what Jesus said about eggs:

"If a son asks for bread from any father among you, will he give him a stone? Or if he asks for a fish, will he give him a serpent instead of a fish? Or if he asks for an egg, will he offer him a scorpion? If you then, being evil, *know how to give good gifts to your chil-*

dren, how much more will your heavenly Father give the Holy Spirit to those who ask Him!" (Luke 11:11–13)

Jesus called eggs "good gifts" to give to our tender children. And they certainly are. Think of what we have in this common little delicacy. An egg is a hygienically-sealed, powerfully packed protein package that can give us a meal in a minute. It can be fried, poached, scrambled, or made into a delicious omelet. If we are hungry, the sound, the sight, and the smell of eggs being fried sends our 10,000 primed tastebuds into a feeding frenzy.

Sue and I have raised chickens and eaten their fresh eggs for more than forty years, and we never get tired of daily collecting these amazing little gifts from Heaven.

The Health Benefits of Eggs

- Eggs contain a high concentration of protein and amino acids. One egg contains 6 grams of protein and all the essential amino acids needed to actually use the protein.

- Due to their high protein and low calories, eggs are great for a weight-loss diet. Protein reduces levels of ghrelin, the hunger hormone, and contributes to feeling satiated. *The Journal of the American College on Nutrition* found out that those who ate eggs for breakfast reduced their overall intake for the next 36 hours. They write, "The egg-breakfast induced greater satiety and significantly reduced short-term food intake."

- Eggs are high in several important nutrients, selenium, vitamin A, phosphorus, riboflavin, and vitamin B12.

- They contain large amounts of omega-3 fatty acids—even non-organic and non-enriched eggs. These acids help to reduce triglycerides in the blood. Omega-3 fatty acids help to relieve inflammation, lower triglycerides, and reduce cholesterol.

- Eggs contain lutein and zeaxanthin, which are important antioxidants that counteract the degenerative processes in the eyes. Cataracts and other common eye disorders can be prevented. Lutein and zeaxanthin also contribute to a healthy skin by filtering harmful blue spectrum rays.

- They contain 300 micrograms of an important micronutrient called choline, which most people don't get enough of. Choline is beneficial for brain and liver functions. In fact, certain brain issues, such as depression and cognitive functions, can be treated with the right amounts of choline.

- They are one of few foods that contain natural vitamin D. (Other sources include certain fish and mushrooms.) Eggs from free-range chickens, which are allowed to roam outdoors, contain significantly more vitamin D than those from chickens kept indoors.

- Eggs can lower the risk of breast cancer by 44% in women who eat at least six eggs a week.

- They contain High Density Lipoprotein (HDL), which is known as good cholesterol. People with good HDL levels can prevent heart disease, strokes, and other health problems. Studies have shown that eating two eggs daily for six weeks can raise HDL levels by 10%. Eggs regulate cholesterol absorption and inflammation in the bloodstream.

- They help reduce the risk of metabolic syndrome, which includes conditions such as heart disease, stroke, and diabetes. One study found that eggs could lower metabolic syndrome and produce a positive, significant impact on blood sugar and triglyceride levels.

- Eggs contain carotenoids, antioxidants that lessen oxidative damage in cells, reducing chronic conditions like diabetes, cancer, and autoimmune disorders.

Sources:

healthfitnessrevolution.com/top-10-benefits-eating-eggs/

draxe.com/nutrition/health-benefits-of-eggs/

pubmed.ncbi.nlm.nih.gov/16373948/

Things to Ponder About the Egg

My good friend Stuart G. Scott is the ultimate egg-lover. Just mention eggs to him and his face lights up with delight. This is what he says about them:

The chicken egg is like a space capsule. It is a self-contained, sealed environment that includes a food supply, a water supply, an oxygen supply, a waste-filtration system, a defense system, and a shock-absorption system—everything the chick needs to grow and survive its twenty-one-day journey into the world.

The shell of an egg contains approximately 10,000 holes. If you place an egg in warm water, you can see tiny lines of bubbles rising from the shell. These holes allow oxygen to enter the capsule and carbon dioxide and waste fluids to exit.

The white of the egg is a gelatin-like substance containing mostly water and some proteins. It acts like a shock absorber for the embryo. The embryo is attached to the outside of the yoke which is suspended in the center of the white by two elastic tethers attached to each end of the capsule. The embryo is further protected by an enzyme in the white called lysozyme. Lysozyme destroys bacteria on contact. It is interesting to note that this same lysozyme is also found in human tears and functions in the same capacity in our immune system: to protect our exposed eyes from bacteria.

As cells in a fertilized egg begin to divide, one of the first things to develop is a network of blood vessels connecting the embryo to the yoke, its food supply, and to the membrane, its oxygen supply and waste-transfer system. These blood vessels become the chick's lifelines.

When an egg is hard boiled and pealed, you notice a membrane around the white of the egg. This membrane is a specialized transfer barrier, allowing the transfer of gases and fluid between the bloodstream and the outside. Oxygen enters the bloodstream and carbon dioxide and waste exit the bloodstream through this transfer mechanism.

On Day 2, the chick's heart is beating and the flow of supplies has begun.

On Day 6, the beak and the egg tooth begin to form and movement starts. The egg tooth is an actual tooth that grows on the *outside* of the chick's beak. It has only one temporary function, but is absolutely necessary. It is the key needed to exit the capsule.

On Day 14 the chick turns its head to the blunt end of the capsule. Have you ever noticed the flat spot on the blunt end of a hard-boiled egg? It is caused by what is called the air sack, which is actually an oxygen supply stored inside the capsule.

On Day 17 the chick turns its beak toward the air sack.

On Day 19 the remaining yoke is drawn into the chick's body, which will sustain the chick for several days after it exits the capsule. At this point the little astronaut is nearly complete.

On Day 21 the chick is ready to hatch. It begins by using its now fully developed egg tooth, the key, and neck muscles to slice into the air sack and start breathing on its own.

The oxygen supply will last for only six hours, though. If the chick does not reach the outside air within six hours, it will die. It somehow knows this and continues to slice the shell with its tooth until it breaks through.

How does the chick know that there is air in the sack? Why doesn't the chick just take it easy once it accesses the air supply and is able to breathe? How does it know how to break out at all? These are specific instructions encoded on its DNA. Where does this information come from?

The chick escapes its little space capsule on exactly day 21 every time. When it emerges, you can often see its lifelines still attached. After a few days it throws the key away and the egg tooth falls off.

Every part just described is absolutely essential. If one part is missing or defective—the 10,000 holes, the specially fitted membrane, the yoke, the white, the enzymes, nutrients, shock absorbers, the egg tooth or neck muscles to break into the reserve air supply—if any of it fails, the entire system fails and we wouldn't have any eggs for breakfast! Each step must take place exactly as it does, at exactly the right time, or there would be no chickens.

How does one account for this by chance? To think that all the information for these processes, instructions, and projects— the materials to use and the structures to build—were all generated from the very dust they are made of is not sane! Add to this the complexity of assembling these parts in their proper order, with the intent of building a self-functioning, self-maintaining, self-diag-nosing, self-repairing, self-replicating machine; then coding, miniaturizing, and packaging all of these instructions on one sperm and one egg, and you remove any pos-sibility of it ever accidentally happening— ever! Yet with one word we can clear up the whole bag of tricks. Design. —Stuart G. Scott, Living Waters Publications

References:

University of Illinois, Incubation and Embryology; Mississippi State University, MSUCares, Poultry; 4H Virtual Farm, Virtual Hatch Project; Dr. Jobe Martin DMD, ThM, *Creatures That Defy Evolution*

TASTEFUL QUOTE
"If you've broken the eggs, you should make the omelette." —Anthony Eden

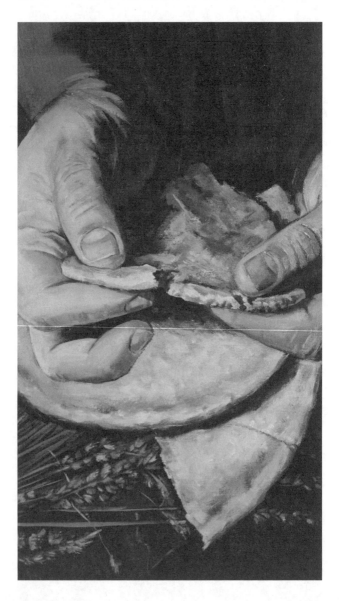

CHAPTER EIGHT

LIFE'S STAPLE DIET

Jesus not only recommended and ate bread, He taught His disciples to ask God for a supply for *daily* consumption:

> "Give us this day our daily bread." (Matthew 6:11)

He also multiplied five loaves to give fresh bread to several thousand hungry souls. When food was needed on another occasion for another few thousand famished folks (see Mark 8:1–10), He miraculously supplied another fresh batch. On both occasions, He made sure not a crumb was wasted:

> When it was evening, His disciples came to Him, saying, "This is a deserted place, and the hour is already late. Send the multitudes away, that they may go into the villages and buy themselves food."

But Jesus said to them, "They do not need to go away. You give them something to eat."

And they said to Him, "We have here only five loaves and two fish."

He said, "Bring them here to Me." Then He commanded the multitudes to sit down on the grass. And He took the five loaves and the two fish, and looking up to heaven, He blessed and broke and gave the loaves to the disciples; and the disciples gave to the multitudes. So they all ate and were filled, *and they took up twelve baskets full of the fragments that remained.* Now those who had eaten were about five thousand men, besides women and children. (Matthew 14:15–21)

The Scriptures say that bread "strengthens man's heart" (Psalm 104:15). *Gill's Exposition of the Entire Bible* says of this verse:

And bread which strengthens man's heart:... bread is made for the support of man's life, and is the chief sustenance of it; and is therefore commonly called "the staff of life", and, by the prophet, "the whole stay of bread", Isaiah 3:1, by which human nature is invigorated, and the strength of man is kept up and increased...Of this nature are the provisions of God's house,...especially Christ Jesus himself, the true and living bread; by which the Christian's spiritual life is supported and maintained, and he is comforted and refreshed, and strengthened for every good work.[26]

Think of one piece of bread as it lies quietly on a plate in front of you. In a sense, it is lifeless. It doesn't walk or talk or think. However, there was a time in the not too distant past when it did have life. As living wheat, it drank water, consumed soil nutrients, absorbed the sunlight, and grew in size.

But as it lies on your plate, it's dead. In time it will become moldy, and then turn to dust. However, as lifeless as it is, it still has the ability not only to taste good and satisfy your hunger, but to put fuel in your tank that can motivate you. Food turns into kinetic energy so that you have the strength to move your body. This is something we so take for granted, the wonder of it hardly enters our minds. Albert Einstein said, "There are only two ways to live your life. One is as though nothing is a miracle. The other is as though everything is a miracle." That's true. Some of us don't like to think about everyday things of life. To see everything (including our food and how it interacts with our body) as the miraculous hand of God will change us from praising what is made to praising the One who made it—where it's justly due.

Another invisible force that we casually call "hunger" causes our wonderfully made eyes to feast on the bread as it lies on the plate. It is our appetite that gives us the desire to eat. Our amazingly dexterous hands pick it up and feed it into our marvelously made and fabulously flexible mouth—where the 10,000 eagerly awaiting tastebuds coordinate with a complex mixture of saturating saliva. All this then combines with the pleasurable chewing process in which our nerve-filled teeth break down the food. Once it's chewed down to the correct size, it's then sent down a pipe into our awaiting stomach—that complex compartment that has the ready and most necessary energy-making machinery.

Think now for a moment of how breathtakingly incredible God is to create all this, not just to give us energy but at the same time give us pleasure:

> All parts of the body (muscles, brain, heart, and liver) need energy to work. This energy comes from the food we eat.
>
> Our bodies digest the food we eat by mixing it with fluids (acids and enzymes) in the stomach. When the stomach digests food, the carbohydrate (sugars and starches) in the food breaks down into another type of sugar, called glucose.
>
> The stomach and small intestines absorb the glucose and then release it into the bloodstream. Once in the bloodstream, glucose can be used immediately for energy or stored in our bodies, to be used later.[27]

Bread in Bible Times

Bread is mentioned nearly five hundred times in the original language of Scripture. It was such a vital part of every meal that the Hebrew word for it, *lehem*, is the same word used to describe their food in general.

The supreme importance of bread to the ancient Israelites is also demonstrated by how Biblical Hebrew has at least a dozen words for bread, and bread features in numerous Hebrew proverbs (for example, Proverbs 20:17, Proverbs 28:19).

Bread was eaten at just about every meal and is estimated to have provided from 50 to 70 percent of an ordinary person's daily calories. The bread eaten until the end of the Israelite monarchy was mainly made from barley flour; during the Second Temple period, bread from wheat flour become predominant.[28]

Health Benefits of Bread

- Whole grain bread is linked to many health benefits. It lowers the risk of heart disease, diabetes, obesity, and colorectal cancer. It is rich in key nutrients such as manganese and selenium.

- Sprouted bread contains more fiber, folate, vitamin E, vitamin C, and beta-carotene but few antinutrients (which can impair the absorption of certain vitamins and minerals). In sprouted grains, the nutrients are more easily digestible and more available to the body for use.

- The American Heart Association notes that whole grains are a good source of B vitamins, including folic acid, iron, magnesium, selenium, and dietary fiber. The AHA recommends at least 25 grams of fiber a day.

- The Harvard T.H. Chan School of Public Health has found that those who eat 70 grams of whole grains per day had a 22% lower risk of premature death, 23% lower risk of death from heart disease, and 20% lower risk of death from cancer, compared to those who consume little or no whole grains. They write, "These findings further support current dietary guidelines that recommend at least 3 daily servings (or 48 grams) of whole grains to improve long-term health and prevent premature death."

Sources:

hsph.harvard.edu/news/press-releases/whole-grains-lower-mortality-rates/

mensjournal.com/food-drink/healthiest-types-bread-and-their-health-benefits/

medicalnewstoday.com/articles/295235#What-is-refined-flour?

TASTEFUL QUOTE
"Here is bread, which strengthens man's heart,
and therefore is called the staff of Life."
—Matthew Henry

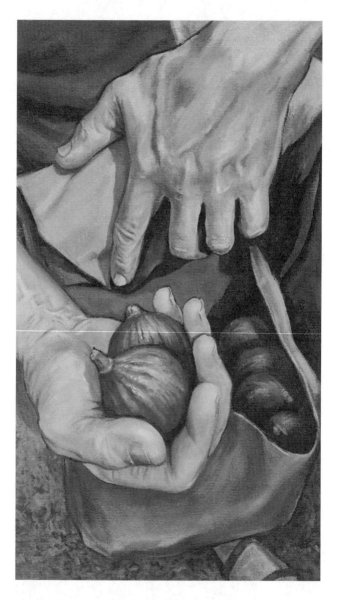

CHAPTER NINE

UNSATISFIED APPETITE

While there is nothing in Scripture about Jesus actually eating figs, there's a strong inference that He did, given to us in two of the four Gospels:

> Now in the morning, as He returned to the city, He was hungry. And seeing a fig tree by the road, He came to it and found nothing on it but leaves, and said to it, "Let no fruit grow on you ever again." Immediately the fig tree withered away. (Matthew 21:18,19)

But is the fact that Jesus *hungered* for figs, and then cursed a tree when it didn't have any, a recommendation for the consumption of figs? Consider that soccer superstar Cristiano Ronaldo once recommended the drinking of water without even taking one sip:

During a Euro 2020 press conference on Monday, soccer superstar Cristiano Ronaldo irritably moved two bottles of Coca-Cola, one of the official sponsors of the event, and then picked up a bottle of water. "Água!" he exclaimed in Portuguese, setting the bottle down in the center of his desk. By the end of the press conference for the European Championships, Coca-Cola's shares had dropped 1.6%, to $55.22 from $56.17. That lopped $4 billion off the beverage behemoth's market value, with the shares sinking another 0.6% on Tuesday to $55.08.[29]

Any food chain is going to leap for joy if a famous person publicly mentions *hungering* after their product. That's a pure gold endorsement that can't be bought.

The fact that Jesus was hungry and wanted to eat figs is a strong recommendation for their consumption. However, there is obviously more here than the shallow thought that Jesus was throwing a temper tantrum because the fig tree had only leaves.

A popular opinion is that the fig tree is a type of national Israel:

This [Jesus cursing the fig tree] is surprising. Until now, Jesus' miracles brought restoration. We cannot say that Jesus acted in frustration. Indeed, Mark 11:13 says, "It was not the season for figs." Still, a fruitful fig tree in the offseason would display small, semi-edible fruits that would later ripen. But this tree was entirely barren. When Jesus cursed it, He performed a symbolic act in the spirit of Jeremiah (Jer. 19:1–11). The fig tree symbolizes Israel. As the fig tree had leaves but no fruit, Israel had a temple, but no spiritual life. Its gleaming buildings teemed with robbery, hypocrisy, and dead ceremony.[30]

And both Matthew and Mark, by "sandwiching" the fig tree episode, focus the lens on where it will all transpire: Jerusalem.

- Matthew: Jerusalem → Fig tree → Jerusalem

- Mark: Fig tree → Jerusalem → Fig tree

Except there's no fruit. The fig tree, once again, has failed. The Passover celebration, the tumult, the crowds, the singing—it's all a show. Jesus enters God's house of prayer and finds it a "den of robbers" (Mark 11:17). Lots of action, lots of bustle, but no righteousness. Leaves, but no fruit.

So upon inspecting the fruitless tree, Jesus pours out divine judgment via two sign-acts: the future-pointing act of cursing the temple, and the enacted metaphor of cursing the tree.[31]

Bible commentator Matthew Henry agrees but goes a little further:

This cursing of the barren fig-tree represents the state of hypocrites in general, and so teaches us that Christ looks for the power of religion in those who profess it, and the savour of it from those that have the show of it. His just expectations from flourishing professors are often disappointed; he comes to many, seeking fruit, and finds leaves only. A false profession commonly withers in this world, and it is the effect of Christ's curse. The fig-tree that had no fruit, soon lost its leaves. This represents the state of the nation and people of the Jews in particular. Our Lord Jesus found among them nothing but leaves. And after they rejected Christ, blindness and hardness grew upon them, till they were undone, and their place and nation rooted up. The Lord was righteous in it. Let us greatly fear the doom denounced on the barren fig-tree.[32]

Perhaps there is also another explanation: that the covering of fig leaves is a type of self-righteousness, the sin that will take multitudes to Hell. We first see it back in Genesis when both Adam and Eve vainly tried to cover themselves with fig leaves as soon as they were conscious of their sin:

> Then the eyes of both of them were opened, and they knew that they were naked; and they sewed fig leaves together and made themselves coverings. (Genesis 3:7)

But the leaves didn't hide their sin, and because of that one act of disobedience, Adam and his descendants came under the curse of God:

> Then to Adam He said, "Because you have heeded the voice of your wife, and have eaten from the tree of which I commanded you, saying, 'You shall not eat of it':
>
> "Cursed is the ground for your sake;
> In toil you shall eat of it
> All the days of your life.
> Both thorns and thistles it shall bring forth for you,
> And you shall eat the herb of the field.
> In the sweat of your face you shall eat bread
> Till you return to the ground,
> For out of it you were taken;
> For dust you are,
> And to dust you shall return." (Genesis 3:17–19)

We cannot escape the curse by our own efforts to keep the moral Law:

> For as many as are of the works of the law are under the curse; for it is written, "Cursed is everyone who does not continue in all things which are written in the book of the law, to do them." (Galatians 3:10)

Jesus spoke about fruitless trees in the Sermon of the Mount:

You will know them by their fruits. Do men gather grapes from thornbushes or figs from thistles? Even so, every good tree bears good fruit, but a bad tree bears bad fruit. A good tree cannot bear bad fruit, nor can a bad tree bear good fruit. Every tree that does not bear good fruit is cut down and thrown into the fire. Therefore by their fruits you will know them. (Matthew 7:16–20)

John the Baptist also spoke against fruitlessness in the lives of professed believers:

And even now the ax is laid to the root of the trees. Therefore every tree which does not bear good fruit is cut down and thrown into the fire. (Matthew 3:10)

In the book of 2 Kings, there is another fig-related story:

In those days Hezekiah was sick and near death. And Isaiah the prophet, the son of Amoz, went to him and said to him, "Thus says the LORD: 'Set your house in order, for you shall die, and not live.'"

Then he turned his face toward the wall, and prayed to the LORD, saying, "Remember now, O LORD, I pray, how I have walked before You in truth and with a loyal heart, and have done what was good in Your sight." And Hezekiah wept bitterly.

And it happened, before Isaiah had gone out into the middle court, that the word of the LORD came to him, saying, "Return and tell Hezekiah the leader of My people, 'Thus says the LORD, the God of David your father: "I have heard your prayer, I have seen your tears; surely I will heal you. On the third day you shall go up to the house of the LORD. And I will add to your days fifteen years. I will deliver you and this city from the hand of the king of Assyria; and I will defend this city for My own sake, and for the sake of My servant David." ' "

Then Isaiah said, "Take a lump of figs." So they took and laid it on the boil, and he recovered. (2 Kings 20:1–7)

The lump of figs that was laid upon the boil was a poultice, as recorded in the book of Isaiah. There it says, "Let them take a lump of figs, and apply it as a poultice on the boil, and he shall recover" (Isaiah 38:21). A poultice is a soft moist mass, often heated, put on cloth and placed on the skin to treat pains or infections.

Figs in Bible Times

Figs were an important source of food. Figs were cultivated throughout the land of Israel, and fresh or dried figs were part of the daily diet. A common way of preparing dried figs was to chop them and press them into a cake. They are one of the biblical Seven Species and are frequently mentioned in the Bible (for example, 1 Samuel 25:18; 1 Samuel 30:12;

and 1 Chronicles 12:41). The remains of dried figs have been discovered from as early as the Neolithic period in Gezer, Israel and Gilgal in the Jordan Valley. The fig tree (*ficus carica*) grew well in the hill country and produced two crops a season. Early-ripening figs were regarded as a delicacy because of their sweetness and were eaten fresh. Figs ripening in the later harvest were often dried and strung into a chain, or pressed into hard round or square-shaped cakes called *develah* and stored as a major source of winter food. The blocks of dried figs were sliced and eaten like bread.[33]

Health Benefits of Figs

- The National Library of Medicine states, "Less than 10% of most Western populations consume adequate levels of whole fruits and dietary fiber with typical intake being about half of the recommended levels. Evidence of the beneficial health effects of consuming adequate levels of whole fruits has been steadily growing, especially regarding their bioactive fiber prebiotic effects and role in improved weight control, wellness and healthy aging."

- Figs are low in calories and make an excellent healthy snack, especially in a weight-loss program. Due to their fiber content, eating two or three figs provides a sensation of satisfaction between meals.

- Figs are rich in copper and vitamin B6, and contain small quantities of a wide variety of nutrients. Copper helps in metabolism, energy production, formation of blood cells, connective tissues, and neurotransmitters. Vitamin B6 is important for the creation of new proteins and for preserving brain health.

- They also promote digestive and heart health by helping to manage blood sugar levels. Fig leaf tea for breakfast decreases the insulin needs of type 1 diabetics. In a 1998 study the insulin doses decreased by 12%. Dried figs, however, are high in sugar and should be eaten in moderation.

- Figs are a good source of calcium and potassium, which work together to improve bone density and prevent conditions like osteoporosis.

- They are rich in fiber, which promotes digestive health by decreasing constipation and working as a prebiotic so that healthy bacteria populate the gut. In animal studies, figs have reduced constipation and improved the symptoms of digestive disorders like ulcerative colitis. Figs are an excellent source of prebiotics.

- Figs are known to reduce stomachache, bloating, and constipation. A study of 150 people with irritable bowel syndrome showed that eating four dried figs (45 grams) twice daily improved symptoms. A similar study using fig paste found that, "F. carica paste supplementation was associated with a significant reduction in colon transit time and a significant improvement in stool type and abdominal discomfort compared with the placebo."

- Some studies have shown that they improve blood pressure and blood fat levels, decreasing the risk of heart disease. Figs are also a great source of antioxidants, which reduce free radicals as well as reduce triglycerides and bad cholesterol.

- In test tube studies, fig leaves have shown to have antitumor activity against human colon cancer, breast cancer, cervical cancer, and liver cancer cells.

- Dried fig fruit has been used to treat dermatitis and other skin conditions like dry and itchy skin as a result of allergies (as with the poultice instructions God gave Isaiah to treat boils). Creams based on dried figs have proven to be more effective than hydrocortisone creams.

- Figs were considered a symbol of fertility in ancient Greece. They have a high iron content, which plays an essential role in the ovulation cycle in women and sperm production in males. Figs are commonly consumed with milk to boost reproductive health.

Sources:

pubmed.ncbi.nlm.nih.gov/30487459/
pubmed.ncbi.nlm.nih.gov/27440682/
healthline.com/nutrition/figs-benefits#benefits
webmd.com/diet/health-benefits-figs#1
pharmeasy.in/blog/6-fantastic-health-benefits-of-fig/

TASTEFUL QUOTE
"Train up a fig tree in the way it should go, and when you are old sit under the shade of it."
—Charles Dickens

CHAPTER TEN

STICKING TO CHICKEN

Late in 2019, I interviewed three students—named Genesis, Brianna, and Joseph—at a local college, asking them about their tastes in food and if they thought there was life after death. The following is a transcript of those conversations.[34]

RAY TO BRIANNA: Is red meat good for you?

BRIANNA: I really don't know.

RAY TO GENESIS: Do you drink milk?

GENESIS: No.

RAY: Butter?

GENESIS: No.

RAY: Eggs?

GENESIS: Every now and then.

RAY: Cheese?

GENESIS: No.

RAY: What do you eat?

GENESIS: I try to stick to chicken.

RAY: Processed chicken?

GENESIS: Yes, unfortunately.

RAY: Are you worried about the pesticides they spray on vegetables?

GENESIS: Yes. There's a lot to be worried about.

RAY TO BRIANNA: Do you eat red meat?

BRIANNA: Yes. I do.

RAY: Chicken?

BRIANNA: Yes.

RAY: Eggs?

BRIANNA: Yes.

RAY: Butter?

BRIANNA: Yes.

RAY: Milk?

BRIANNA: Yes.

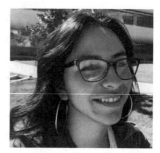

Brianna

RAY: You're not worried about what you eat, and you're probably more healthy than someone who is worrying themselves to death.

GENESIS: (Laughs.)

RAY: Genesis, do you believe there's an afterlife?

GENESIS: Yes, I do.

BRIANNA: I think it just comforts me, knowing that this isn't all there is to it.

RAY: Are you afraid of dying?

BRIANNA: I don't know. I like to think I'm not, but I am. It's like, if I died right now, I'd be kind of scared.

GENESIS: I'm comfortable with knowing that, okay, eventually we all get to that point, but—

RAY: What point?

GENESIS: To where we have to die.

RAY: Why? Ever wonder why? Everything dies. Your puppy dies, your grandma dies, grandpa dies. Your mom and dad die, you're going to die. Why? Do you believe in God?

GENESIS: I'm trying.

RAY TO BRIANNA: You believe in God?

BRIANNA: I do.

RAY: There's actually a way to know God exists, very simply. Did you know that?

BRIANNA: No.

RAY TO GENESIS: Did you know that?

GENESIS: Tell me.

RAY: It's very simple. When you look at a building, you don't *believe* there was a builder, you *know* there was a builder. He could have died a hundred years ago, but you know somebody built it because buildings don't build themselves. Exactly the same applies with paintings and painters. You look at a painting, you don't *believe* there was a painter, you *know* there was a painter, because paintings can't paint themselves; it's impossible. If the painter had died two thousand years ago, you'd still know there was a painter, because of the fact that paintings can't paint themselves. So, when you look at creation, you know intuitively that there is a Creator; it's common sense.

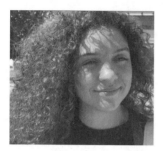

Genesis

It's impossible for nature to make itself. You've got flowers, birds, trees, sun, moon, stars, puppies, kittens, ponies, lambs, chickens—in all these things we see the genius of God's creative hand. Because man, with all his genius, can't even make a grain of sand from nothing. So it's crazy to think that nothing created everything from an explosion in space that gave us all these wonderful things we see around us. Do you realize that we're feeling the warmth of the sun at the moment? It's kind of nice—it's warm. It's coming from 93 million miles away. If it was just a little bit closer, we would die. So everything has order to it. You know, all around us, we see order—from the atom to the universe—which tells us we're intelligently designed.

RAY TO JOSEPH: Do you think God's happy with you or angry at you, Joseph?

JOSEPH: That's a very good question that I've been thinking about lately. I feel like God is in between happy and angry. Like, He's given me days to live, but, at the same time, He's a little angry at me, because I feel like He's punished me lately. And He wants me to wake up because I've been doing things that are not really, in a way, like, good.

RAY: Are you a good person?

JOSEPH: I do consider myself a good person.

RAY: Okay, I'm going to see if I can change your mind on that. Do you know what a paradigm shift is?

JOSEPH: A paradigm shift? No.

RAY: A paradigm shift. Let me give you one. A man who was blind got onto a bus, and someone stood up and gave him a seat. Was that a good thing to do?

JOSEPH: Yes, that's a good thing to do.

RAY: It's actually very bad; that guy lost his job for doing it. You know why?

JOSEPH: Why is that?

RAY: He was the bus driver.

JOSEPH: Oh, haha.

RAY: That's a paradigm shift. I gave you information that radically changed your mind. You went from, "That's a good thing," to "Woah, that's a bad thing." So information is very powerful. I'm going to give you information that I think's going to change you and your attitude about yourself when it comes to God. So you think you're a good person?

JOSEPH: Yes.

RAY: How many lies have you told in your life?

JOSEPH: Countless.

RAY: What do you call someone who tells many lies?

JOSEPH: A liar.

RAY: So what are you?

JOSEPH: A liar.

RAY: Now do you still think you're a good person?

JOSEPH: (Laughs.)

RAY: Isn't it hard to say about yourself? You know, if someone tells countless lies, he's a liar, but when it comes to ourselves, it's really hard to judge ourselves. It's like bad breath. It takes an objective person like a girlfriend or a wife to say, "Honey, your breath stinks. You need to do something," or, "You need to change your clothes, you've got body odor." It takes an outward source to do that, and it's the same with us morally. Have you ever stolen something in your life, even if it's small?

JOSEPH: Have I ever stolen something in my life? Yes, I have.

RAY: So what are you?

JOSEPH: A thief.

RAY: No, you're a lying thief.

JOSEPH: Oh, ha. I'm a lying thief.

RAY: Have you ever used God's name in vain?

JOSEPH: Yes.

RAY: Would you use your mother's name as a cuss word?

JOSEPH: I would never.

RAY: Because you'd dishonor her—it'd be a horrible thing to do.

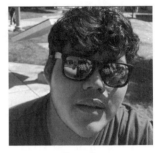

Joseph

And yet, God gave you eyes to see with, ears to hear good music with, a brain to think with, tastebuds to enjoy good food. He lavished His kindness upon you, and you took His holy name and used it to cuss, which is called blasphemy. Punishable by death in the Old Testament. This is not comfortable, but stay with me, because it's worth it. Jesus said, "If you look at a woman and lust for her, you commit adultery with her in your heart." Have you ever looked at a woman with lust?

JOSEPH: Yes, I have.

RAY: Have you had sex before marriage?

JOSEPH: Yes, I have.

RAY: So, Joseph, I'm not judging you, but you've just told me you're a lying, thieving, blasphemous, fornicating adulterer at heart. Do you still think you're a good person?

JOSEPH: Yes, I do, in a way.

RAY: How could you think a lying thief is a good person? I'll tell you how: your standard of judgment is very low. God's is very high. If you look up the word "good" in the dictionary, there are over forty different definitions. Number one is "moral excellence," and none of us are morally excellent. So you're in big trouble on Judgment Day; can you see that?

JOSEPH: Yes, I am.

RAY: Would you go to Heaven or Hell if you're found guilty on that Day?

JOSEPH: I'd go to Hell.

RAY: So, does that concern you?

JOSEPH: In a way, it does.

RAY: Let me tell you what the Scripture says. It says all liars will have their part in the Lake of Fire. No thief, no adulterer, no blasphemer will inherit God's Kingdom. So you're in big trouble. Do you know what the Bible actually says? It says that we're enemies of God in our mind through wicked works. And there's no greater evidence that we're enemies of God than that we use His name as a cuss word. And every time we sin, we store up His wrath that's going to be revealed on the Day of Judgment. Do you know what death is? It's punishment from God for sin. The Bible says, "The wages of sin is death." Ever wonder what it would be like to be on death row? Found guilty and waiting to be executed—wouldn't that be horrible?

JOSEPH: Yes, it would be horrible, yeah.

RAY: You'd be in a cell, tormented by the fact that you're getting closer and closer to being executed. That's where you and I are. We've got a nice big holding cell, beautiful blue roof, good lighting, good air conditioning, but this life is a holding cell. We're waiting to be executed, because we've sinned against God. Death will seize upon us, drag us before the Judge of the universe, to answer for violating His Law. And Hell is God's prison, and there's no parole.

Now, Christian background. What did God do for guilty sinners so we wouldn't have to go to Hell? Do you remember? Let me tell you. He sent a Savior. Jesus suffered and died on the cross. You and I violated God's Law, the Ten

Commandments. Jesus came and paid the fine. *That's* what happened on that cross. That's why Jesus said, "It is finished," just before He died. In other words, the debt has been paid. Joseph, if you're in court and someone pays your fine, the judge can let you go, even though you're guilty. He can say, "Joseph, there's a stack of speeding fines here, this is deadly serious. But someone's paid them—you're free to go," and he can do that which is legal and right and just. And God can *legally* dismiss your case, forgive all those sins in an instant, and let you live forever, legally, because of what Jesus did on the cross: paying the fine in His life's blood, and then rising from the dead and defeating death.

And if you'll repent—not just confess your sins to a priest, but actually repent before God, and repentance means to turn from sin, acknowledge it and turn from it—[He will forgive you]. Don't say, "I'm a Christian," and you lie, steal, fornicate, look at pornography; that's just deceiving yourself. So you've got to be genuine in your repentance. And secondly, you must trust in Jesus, like you'd trust a parachute. Let me give you a quick analogy, and then I'll let you go. If I put you over the edge of a thousand-foot cliff, right on the edge, with your toes over and the stones crumbling beneath your feet, would that be scary for you?

JOSEPH: Yes, it would be.

RAY: Would the feeling of fear be a good feeling or a bad feeling?

JOSEPH: It'd be a good feeling.

RAY: No, it wouldn't, it'd be terrifying!

JOSEPH: Well, yes it would, but it'd show you how close you are to death.

RAY: That's exactly right, that's where I was going next. You jumped the gun a little. The feeling would be horrible, but the fear itself would be good because it's doing you a favor. It's saying, "Back up, back up! You're in danger!" So, your fear is your friend, not your enemy. What I've tried to do with you, and it's been uncomfortable, a horrible feeling, is hang you over the cliff of eternity by your feet, just for a few minutes, so you'll feel fear in the fact that you've sinned against God. The Bible says that the fear of the Lord is the beginning of wisdom; through the fear of the Lord, men depart from sin. So, I want you to see that feeling, that horrible feeling, as your friend, not your enemy, because it's showing you you're in danger, eternal danger of being damned by God, of dying in your sins and getting justice. That's a horrific thought.

RAY TO BRIANNA: Upon conversion, God will change your heart so that you love that which is right. That's your own personal miracle from God. So are you going to think about what we talked about?

BRIANNA: Yes.

RAY: Seriously?

BRIANNA: Yes.

RAY: Do you have a Bible at home?

BRIANNA: I do.

RAY: And do you?

GENESIS: Yes.

RAY: Ladies, it's been an honor to speak with you. I've really appreciated the fact that you've been patient with me, and you've listened intently, and I trust that you will seriously think about this. Nice to meet you.

GENESIS AND BRIANNA: You too.

RAY TO JOSEPH: I love you and I care about you, and the thought of you ending up in Hell would horrify me. So, are you going to think about this?

JOSEPH: Yes, I will.

RAY: You going to seriously think about it?

JOSEPH: Serious in what way?

RAY: Well, if you were on the edge of a thousand-foot cliff, you could say, "This is dangerous, I'm going to think about this," or you can say, "This is dangerous, I'm stepping back *right now*." That's what I want you to do, to turn from sin and trust in the Savior, because you could die today—150,000 people die every 24 hours. So can you see what I'm saying?

JOSEPH: Yes, I do.

RAY: The thing that'll stop you coming to Christ is your love for sin. Pornography and fornication are incredibly pleasurable to the sinful human heart. We just love sin, the Bible says that. We love darkness rather than light because our deeds are evil. But the miracle of conversion is that God will give you a new heart with new desires. The moment you repent and trust the Savior, you'll be born again, and you'll love that which is right, and that's a personal miracle. You'll say, "Man, I don't want to do what's wrong, I want to do what's right." It's radical when that happens. Like I said, it's your personal miracle. You don't need to see visions, all you need is a changed heart that loves God and wants to serve Him with every ounce of energy you've got, because He is the one who gave you life. Does that make sense?

JOSEPH: Yes, it does.

RAY: You gonna think seriously about this?

JOSEPH: Yes, I will.

RAY: Do you have a Bible at home?

JOSEPH: I think…yes, I do have a Bible at home.

RAY: Would you be embarrassed if I pray for you?

JOSEPH: No.

RAY: Father, I thank you for Joseph, and his open heart today. I pray that you would give him a new heart with new desires. May he be born again and love you and serve you, and be a light to this generation. In Jesus' name we pray, amen.

JOSEPH: Amen.

CHAPTER ELEVEN

AFTER BREAKFAST

In the previous chapters, we have looked at the nine foods that Jesus either consumed or recommended. They are butter, honey, fish, lamb, veal, salt, eggs, bread, and figs. These are foods that without question are good for our health. But sadly, each of us will still die even if we live a long life in the best of health. This is why we need the spiritual food of which Jesus spoke—the food that leads to everlasting life.

It was immediately *after* the bread and fish breakfast (see John 21:12) that Jesus spoke to Peter about the importance of feeding his brethren spiritual food. It isn't wise for a husband and wife to discuss finances or talk about some problem before they eat a meal. This is because we are often agitated when we're hungry. Whenever I traveled by plane and wanted to share the gospel with someone sitting next to me, I would almost always wait until after they had eaten their meal. Jesus did the same thing with Peter:

> So when they had eaten breakfast, Jesus said to Simon Peter, "Simon, son of Jonah, do you love Me more than these?"
>
> He said to Him, "Yes, Lord; You know that I love You."
>
> He said to him, "Feed My lambs."
>
> He said to him again a second time, "Simon, son of Jonah, do you love Me?"
>
> He said to Him, "Yes, Lord; You know that I love You."
>
> He said to him, "Tend My sheep."
>
> He said to him the third time, "Simon, son of Jonah, do you love Me?" Peter was grieved because He said to him the third time, "Do you love Me?"
>
> And he said to Him, "Lord, You know all things; You know that I love You."
>
> Jesus said to him, "Feed My sheep." (John 21:15–17)

While the world ignores this spiritual food, we can see its essential nature, in that Jesus emphasized its importance three times in three different ways, just in this one occasion.

Food at the Forefront

Eating was at the front and center of the greatest of all human tragedies. Every terrible human suffering, all frightening killer diseases, and even the horror of death itself traces back to this one incident:

> Now the serpent was more cunning than any beast of the field which the LORD God had made. And he said to the woman, "Has God indeed said, 'You shall not eat of every tree of the garden'?"
>
> And the woman said to the serpent, "We may eat the fruit of the trees of the garden; but of the fruit of the tree which is in the midst of the garden, God has said, 'You shall not eat it, nor shall you touch it, lest you die.'"
>
> Then the serpent said to the woman, "You will not surely die. For God knows that in the day you eat of it your eyes will be opened, and you will be like God, knowing good and evil."
>
> So when the woman saw that the tree was good for food, that it was pleasant to the eyes, and a tree desirable to make one wise, she took of its fruit and ate. She also gave to her husband with her, and he ate. Then the eyes of both of them were opened, and they knew that they were naked; and they sewed fig leaves together and made themselves coverings. (Genesis 3:1–6)

The New Testament gives us further insight into this event by telling us that Eve was a victim of deception. She was deceived by the craftiness of the serpent (2 Corinthians 11:3). However, Adam *wasn't* deceived. He went into sin with his eyes wide open: "And Adam was not deceived, but the woman being deceived, fell into transgression" (1 Timothy 2:14).

And so Adam is forever held responsible for sin and suffering, disease and death:

> Therefore, just as through one man sin entered the world, and death through sin, and thus death spread to all men, because all sinned. (Romans 5:12)

Like Eve, we were also once deceived by the god of this world who blinded our minds to the gospel (see 2 Corinthians 4:3,4). Scripture tells us, "For we ourselves were also once foolish, disobedient, deceived, serving various lusts and pleasures, living in malice and envy, hateful and hating one another" (Titus 3:3).

And so (until we come to Christ), each of us is found in the unenviable position of being enemies of God, under His curse, and helplessly heading for death and damnation:

> For if when we were enemies we were reconciled to God through the death of His Son, much more, having been reconciled, we shall be saved by His life. (Romans 5:10)

In this fallen world, whether we live or die depends on our consumption of *physical* food. And whether we live in the next life depends on our consumption of *spiritual* food. When Jesus was gripped by near starvation after fasting for forty days, Satan tempted Him to turn stones into bread. Surely turning stones into bread wouldn't have been sinful. He was close to dying of hunger; bread would save His life. But consider what Jesus said:

> "It is written, 'Man shall not live by bread alone, but by every word that proceeds from the mouth of God.'" (Matthew 4:4)

There is a spiritual food that nourishes our soul, and it comes to us directly from God. In John 6, there is an intense discourse on the subject of this spiritual food. After Jesus multiplied the loaves, a crowd followed Him because they were so thoroughly satisfied by the complimentary bread and fish lunch:

> Jesus answered them and said, "Most assuredly, I say to you, you seek Me, not because you saw the signs, but because you ate of the loaves and were filled." (John 6:26)

As we were before God opened the eyes of our understanding, they were only interested in natural food. But Jesus introduced them to the supernatural food—that one that comes out of the mouth of God. He said,

> "Do not labor for the food which perishes, but for the food which endures to everlasting life, which the Son of Man will give you,

because God the Father has set His seal on Him."

Then they said to Him, "What shall we do, that we may work the works of God?"

Jesus answered and said to them, "This is the work of God, that you believe in Him whom He sent."

Therefore they said to Him, "What sign will You perform then, that we may see it and believe You? What work will You do? Our fathers ate the manna in the desert; as it is written, 'He gave them bread from heaven to eat.'" (John 6:27–31)

The Pharisees wanted a sign that Jesus was from God, and they pointed to a time in their history in which bread was supernaturally supplied from Heaven. But they wrongly believed that Moses was the miracle-worker:

Then Jesus said to them, "Most assuredly, I say to you, Moses did not give you the bread from heaven, but My Father gives you the true bread from heaven. For the bread of God is He who comes down from heaven and gives life to the world."

Then they said to Him, "Lord, give us this bread always."

And Jesus said to them, "I am the bread of life. He who comes to Me shall never hunger, and he who believes in Me shall never thirst." (John 6:32–35)

Think about what Jesus is claiming. He said that He was the preexistent source of all life—*that He came down from Heaven!* The Jews heard Him say that, and they were offended:

> The Jews then complained about Him, because He said, "I am the bread which came down from heaven." And they said, "Is not this Jesus, the son of Joseph, whose father and mother we know? How is it then that He says, 'I have come down from heaven'?" ...
>
> "Most assuredly, I say to you, he who believes in Me has everlasting life. I am the bread of life. Your fathers ate the manna in the wilderness, and are dead. This is the bread which comes down from heaven, that one may eat of it and not die. I am the living bread which came down from heaven. If anyone eats of this bread, he will live forever; and the bread that I shall give is My flesh, which I shall give for the life of the world." (John 6:41,42,47–51)

His words force us to make some sort of conclusion. Was this Man from God, or was He delusional? Someone who is delusional is "characterized by or holding idiosyncratic beliefs or impressions that are contradicted by reality or rational argument, typically as a symptom of mental disorder." Jesus fit that bill. So there is no fence upon which to sit. Either this was God telling us how to find everlasting life—and we should listen to Him with undivided attention—or He was insane, and therefore should be completely ignored. But it gets worse. Listen to what He then said:

> The Jews therefore quarreled among themselves, saying, "How can this Man give us His flesh to eat?"
>
> Then Jesus said to them, "Most assuredly, I say to you, unless you eat the flesh of the Son of Man and drink His blood, you have no life in you. Whoever eats My flesh and drinks My blood has eternal life, and I will raise him up at the last day. For My flesh is food indeed, and My blood is drink indeed. He who eats My flesh and drinks My blood abides in Me, and I in him. As the living Father sent Me, and I live because of the Father, so he who feeds on Me will live because of Me. This is the bread which came down from heaven—not as your fathers ate the manna, and are dead. He who eats this bread will live forever." (John 6:52–58)

What did Jesus mean about being the bread which came down from Heaven? And what did He mean about eating His flesh and drinking His blood, and consequently living forever? The answers are found in what He said when He instituted the Last Supper:

> And He took bread, gave thanks and broke it, and gave it to them, saying, "This is My body

which is given for you; do this in remembrance of Me." (Luke 22:19)

For I received from the Lord that which I also delivered to you: that the Lord Jesus on the same night in which He was betrayed took bread; and when He had given thanks, He broke it and said, "Take, eat; this is My body which is broken for you; do this in remembrance of Me." (1 Corinthians 11:23,24)

Notice that the Lord's Supper was instituted as a reminder of what Jesus did on the cross. He said, "This is My body which is broken for you; *do this in remembrance of Me.*" That's the reason we take the bread and wine during communion. His body was broken and His blood shed for us at the cross. He wasn't saying that He was literal bread and we were to literally eat His flesh:

When He called the bread His body, Jesus was physically present with His disciples, His body unbroken. How could He have been offering His broken body to His disciples the night *before* He died? Jesus often spoke in metaphors, calling Himself the door, the shepherd, the vine, etc. He was speaking metaphorically on this occasion, as well.[35]

Look at what Jesus Himself said of His words after many of His disciples were offended by such foolish talk:

Therefore many of His disciples, when they heard this, said, "This is a hard saying; who can understand it?"

When Jesus knew in Himself that His disciples complained about this, He said to them, "Does this offend you? What then if you should see the Son of Man ascend where He was before? It is the Spirit who gives life; the flesh profits nothing. The words that I speak to you are spirit, and they are life." (John 6:60–63)

His words weren't to be taken literally. He said, "The words that I speak to you are spirit, and they are life." They weren't literal statements; they were *spiritual* words. But many, who didn't understand that, took them literally and left Him:

From that time many of His disciples went back and walked with Him no more. Then Jesus said to the twelve, "Do you also want to go away?"

But Simon Peter answered Him, "Lord, to whom shall we go? You have the words of eternal life. Also we have come to believe and know that You are the Christ, the Son of the living God." (John 6:66–69)

When Jesus spoke so earnestly to Peter after the bread and fish breakfast, He was in essence emphasizing the importance of first being born of the Spirit and then living in the Spirit:

But you are not in the flesh but in the Spirit, if indeed the Spirit of God dwells in you. Now if anyone does not have the Spirit of Christ, he is not His. And if Christ is in you, the body is dead because of sin, but the Spirit is life because of righteousness. But if the Spirit of Him who raised Jesus from the dead dwells in you, He who raised Christ from the dead will also give life to your mortal bodies through His Spirit who dwells in you. (Romans 8:9–11)

TASTEFUL QUOTE
"What nicer thing can you do for somebody than make them breakfast?"
—Anthony Bourdain

CHAPTER TWELVE

DIVINE DINING

One of the greatest evidences that the Bible is God's Word is prophecy. Only God knows the future, and He gave us certain signs to look for so that we would know the time of His coming Kingdom— when His will will be done on earth as it is in Heaven.

One of the greatest of these signs is the Jews obtaining Jerusalem (see Luke 21:24), and then becoming a big problem for all the nations (see Zechariah 12:3). They obtained Jerusalem in 1967, and since then the city has become an excruciating political headache for the United Nations. (For more details, see *Counting the Days* by Ray Comfort.)

More of these signs are listed in the first book of Timothy. They are:

- A falling away from the faith
- Interest in the occult
- Lying
- Hypocrisy
- Immorality
- A forsaking of holy matrimony (the marriage of one man and one woman)
- Commanding to abstain from certain foods:

> Now the Spirit expressly says that in latter times some will depart from the faith, giving heed to deceiving spirits and doctrines of demons, speaking lies in hypocrisy, having their own conscience seared with a hot iron, forbidding to marry, and commanding to abstain from foods which God created to be received with thanksgiving by those who believe and know the truth. For every creature of God is good, and nothing is to be refused if it is received with thanksgiving; for it is sanctified by the word of God and prayer. (1 Timothy 4:1–5)

As we have seen, commanding people to abstain from certain foods is certainly prevalent in contemporary society. The "experts" have vilified eggs, cheese, white meat, dark meat, red meat, milk, butter, honey, bread, potatoes, trans fats, carbs, grains, fruits, cakes, corn syrup, hydrogenated vegetable oil, cookies, tomatoes, fries, nuts, and rice—for starters.

If it's boiled, baked, or fried, it's no good. For every expert who tells you these things are good, ten will tell you they're bad.

The Scriptures warn us about the error of taking advice from this fallen world:

> Blessed [fortunate, prosperous, and favored by God] is the man who does not walk in the counsel of the wicked [following their advice and example]… (Psalm 1:1, AMP)

We can either skate on the thin ice of advice from a world that strains at gnats and swallows camels, or we trust in the solidity of God's Word for what is good to eat. To use a popular idiom, we should take what this world says about food "with a grain of salt."

For the last twenty or so years, I have cooked most of our meals. I have a home office and get great pleasure in having a cooked meal ready for Sue, after she's done a full day's work at our ministry. Each meal has a variety of steamed vegetables. I steam them because steaming retains their nutrients:

> "From 20 to 50 percent of the vitamins, minerals and healthy plant matter can go down the drain with the used water if the vegetables are boiled," says Grethe Iren Borge, a senior researcher at the Norwegian Institute of Food, Fisheries and Aquaculture Research

... "If you steam the vegetables instead, you reduce this loss by half."[36]

Look at these interesting verses about vegetables, from the book of Daniel:

> So Daniel said to the steward whom the chief of the eunuchs had set over Daniel, Hananiah, Mishael, and Azariah, "Please test your servants for ten days, and let them give us vegetables to eat and water to drink. Then let our appearance be examined before you, and the appearance of the young men who eat the portion of the king's delicacies; and as you see fit, so deal with your servants." So he consented with them in this matter, and tested them ten days.
>
> And at the end of ten days their features appeared better and fatter in flesh than all the young men who ate the portion of the king's delicacies. Thus the steward took away their portion of delicacies and the wine that they were to drink, and gave them vegetables. (Daniel 1:11–16)

I serve meat for protein, have salt at the meal to bring out the taste, and put a smidge of butter on the vegetables to give them even more flavor. We eat plenty of home-grown eggs, tasty figs, delicious fish, and of course daily butter and honey on toast at breakfast. We also eat the popular "Ezekiel bread," which is based on Ezekiel 4:9 to create unrivaled nutrition: "Also take for yourself wheat, barley, beans, lentils, millet, and spelt; put them into one vessel, and make bread of them for yourself." The following is from the bread maker's website:

> It's this special, unique combination of 6 grains and legumes that harvests benefits beyond what we normally expect from our breads, pastas, cereals, and other foods.
>
> - Source of Complete Protein – Rated 84.3% as efficient as the highest source of protein (comparable to that of milk or eggs)
> - Contains 18 Amino Acids – Including all 9 essential amino acids
> - Increased Digestibility – Sprouting breaks down starches in grains into simple sugars so your body can digest them easily.
> - Increased Absorption of Minerals – Sprouting breaks down enzyme inhibitors, so your body can more easily absorb calcium, magnesium, iron, copper and zinc.
> - Increased Vitamin C – Sprouting produces vitamin C.
> - Increased Vitamin B – Sprouting increases the vitamin B2, B5 & B6.
> - Great Source of Fiber – Combining sprouted grains and legumes gives a good amount of natural fiber in each serving.[37]

We also eat dark chocolate every day. Here is one time that I unquestioningly listen to the experts. They say that it contains an antioxidant called theobromine, which helps to boost the immune system by protecting the body's cells from free radicals. According to research, theobromine may also help protect the heart, by increasing blood flow, lowering blood pressure, reducing "bad" cholesterol and improving "good" cholesterol. A study of elderly men showed that it reduced the risk of death from heart disease by 50% over a fifteen-year period. It also improves cognitive function and boosts energy and mood.[38]

If these experts happen to change their minds and say they've discovered that dark chocolate isn't good after all, I will ignore them. Mainly because of the following:

> Jeanne Calment lived to be 122 years, five months, and 14 days old. She attributed her long life and youthful glow to her diet and active lifestyle. Every day of her old age, roughly from age 85 onward, she would wake at 6:45 a.m. and start her day with prayer. Until she was 116 years old, she'd finish all meals with a dessert, usually eating about two pounds of chocolate per week.[39]

The dear lady downed *two pounds* of chocolate every week. God bless her.

One other food confession. I take my grandchildren out to lunch on Fridays for fast-food. They order hamburgers, and all I get is one bag of fries. It's a very special time for me. There are some things in life for a grandparent that really make it worth living. During the week I find myself looking forward to the moment I see those cute little salt-covered fries.

Divine Dinner (for two)

I created a basic meal—solely using the nine foods highlighted in this book—and sent it to New York chef Lance Nitahara for his professional touch. Lance is the winner of the Food Network's *Iron Chef* and *Chopped* competitions, as well as numerous other awards, including the ACF Gold Medal, 2006 New York Salon of Culinary Art, New York City, and the ACF Gold Medal, 2012 John Joyce Culinary Challenge.

Here are the recipes for a healthy, biblically based meal for two to nourish our body.

APPETIZER | Crispy Roasted Tilapia

Ingredients:

2 tilapia fillets[40] (approx. 3 oz. each)

3 oz. unleavened bread, such as pita bread or matzo cracker

1 whole egg, beaten

Salt to taste

Instructions:

1. Preheat oven to 375° F.

2. Grind bread or matzo in a food processor or chop fine with a knife.

3. Lay tilapia fillets on a baking sheet and brush with beaten egg.

4. Season with salt and sprinkle ground bread meal over fish until well covered.

5. Bake until fish is cooked through and crust is crispy and golden brown, about 6–8 minutes. Serve hot.

ENTRÉE | Veal and Lamb Omelet

Ingredients:

3 whole eggs

2 oz. butter

2 oz. veal shoulder, cut into 1/2-inch cubes

2 boneless lamb chops, about 1/2-inch thick

Salt to taste

Instructions:

1. Melt 1/2 oz. butter in a non-stick pan until foaming. Season veal shoulder with salt and cook over medium-high heat until well browned on all sides. Add water to pan, enough to cover the veal halfway, and bring to a simmer. Cook until tender, about 10 minutes. Remove from pan and shred with a fork. Reserve.

2. Add 1/2 oz. butter to same pan, season, and cook lamb chops about 3 minutes per side until well browned but still pink in the center. (The temperature in the center should measure about 130° F.) Reserve.

3. Add 1 oz. butter to pan and melt until foaming. While the butter is melting, crack the eggs into a bowl and whisk well. Season with salt. Add shredded veal to the pan, cook briefly, then add the eggs. Stir until a wet scrambled egg consistency has been achieved and then spread egg out across the pan.

4. Remove from heat and lay the lamb chops, shingled, across the omelet. Fold omelet over and slide onto a plate. If preferred, cut in half and place on two plates. Garnish with parsley or an olive leaf.

DESSERT | Honey-Glazed Figs

Ingredients:
6 fresh figs
2 oz. honey

Instructions:

1. Preheat oven to 375° F.

2. Line a baking pan with parchment paper. Cut figs in half and place them cut side up on the pan.

3. Drizzle figs with honey.

4. Bake for 20 minutes until they bubble and are lightly caramelized. Serve warm.

Back to Timothy

The book of Timothy then goes on to speak of the nourishment that is more important than our physical food. It is the importance of being "nourished in the words of faith and of the good doctrine":

> If you instruct the brethren in these things, you will be a good minister of Jesus Christ, nourished in the words of faith and of the good doctrine which you have carefully followed. But reject profane and old wives' fables, and exercise yourself toward godliness. For bodily exercise profits a little, but godliness is profitable for all things, having promise of the life that now is and of that which is to come. (1 Timothy 4:6–8)

Once again, Scripture clashes with the experts of this world who tell us to daily run, walk, lift, and sweat our heart out as if our life depends on it. The Bible says that bodily exercise profits "a little." So do your exercises, but write this on the inside of your sweating bow: "Bodily exercise profits a little, but *godliness is profitable for all things*, having promise of the life that now is and of that which is to come."

In the next chapter we will look at what we can do to boost our immune system—the things we should all have on our to-do list.

CHAPTER THIRTEEN

BOOSTING YOUR IMMUNE SYSTEM

Every sane person wants to live a long and healthy life, so I have collected twelve keys on how to best do that—many of which are just common sense. With each one, I've added ways we can boost our spiritual immune system. The first is obvious.

1. Don't smoke.

Breathing any form of smoke into our precious lungs is not only deadly for our health, it's foolish. If we were in a room that suddenly filled with smoke, we would immediately run outside to get fresh air, put on a mask, or at least open windows to let in fresh air. But the thoughtless cigarette smoker habitually breathes multiple deadly poisons *in concentrated form* into his lungs, polluting his blood, his brain, and his lungs with every breath. What he does is equivalent to a man who has a bad habit of repeatedly poking his eyeballs with a tiny needle—because it gives him some sort of twisted pleasure. He says that it seems like a crazy thing to do, but after a while you get used to it and it doesn't cause too much pain. He can only blame himself when he goes blind.

Once we come to the Savior, we discover that sin is a perverted and poisonous pleasure that should be avoided at all costs. Jesus said, "And if your eye causes you to sin, pluck it out and cast it from you. It is better for you to enter into life with one eye, rather than having two eyes, to be cast into hell fire" (Matthew 18:9). Enjoyable though it may be, sin will eventually pay terrible wages to all those who serve it—because its payment is death (see Romans 6:23). Scripture gives us a window of fresh air to get rid of the destructive behavior of serving sin:

> Finally, brethren, whatever things are true, whatever things are noble, whatever things are just, whatever things are pure, whatever things are lovely, whatever things are of good report, if there is any virtue and if there is anything praiseworthy—meditate on these things. (Philippians 4:8)

2. Eat a diet high in fruits and vegetables.
There are certain foods that most nutritionists suggest that we eat. But there is unanimous agreement that we should eat *plenty* of vegetables—three to

five cups per day, or more. Broccoli, for example, is supercharged with vitamins A, C, and E, and sweet potatoes are rich in beta carotene.

Discipline yourself to feed on the Word of God every day. It is supercharged with spiritual vitamins. Psalm 1 promises our continued health if we chew it over daily. Say to yourself, "No Bible, no breakfast. No read, no feed," and you'll never go wrong—if you stick to that diet.

3. Exercise regularly.

Our body is a sophisticated machine that should be maintained with the oil of regular exercise. Whatever the particular exercise, experts suggest that it's helpful to push the intensity or pace for a minute or two, then back off for anywhere from two to ten minutes, and to continue doing this throughout the workout. Again, it does have profit, but just a little.

> But have nothing to do with irreverent folklore and silly myths. On the other hand, discipline yourself for the purpose of godliness [keeping yourself spiritually fit]. For physical training is of some value, but godliness (spiritual training) is of value in everything and in every way, since it holds promise for the present life and for the life to come. This is a faithful and trustworthy saying worthy of full acceptance and approval. (1 Timothy 4:7–9, AMP)

4. Maintain a healthy weight.

If we refuse to exercise self-control when it comes to the monster of appetite, we will eventually be overcome by it. Being overweight can be deadly, because it can cause serious health issues.

However, the soul is different. The Scriptures tell us, "Let your soul delight itself in fatness" (Isaiah 55:2, KJV). When we love God we will feast on His Word. He prepares a table for us in the presence of our enemies, and as we take in the Word of God, our soul will become delightfully plump with love, gentleness, goodness, and kindness.

5. Avoid alcohol.

The world says that if we do drink alcohol, we should drink only in moderation. But when someone has too much alcohol, they are said to be "intoxicated." The word "intoxicate" comes from the Latin *intoxicare*, meaning "to poison."

This poison leaves a trail of destruction—including causing blackouts, slurred speech, brain shrinkage, dependence, heart damage, liver damage, pancreatitis, heart damage, liver damage, infertility, sexual dysfunction, behavioral changes, cancer, thinning of bones, muscle cramps, and lung infections.[41]

Yet the world can't bring itself to say, "Don't drink alcohol." This is because it loves its benefit. It temporarily dulls the human conscience. It gives men the boldness to follow their sinful passions, and it softens a woman's intuitive resistance to sexual sin. Many a virtuous woman has tragically lost her virtue because of the deception of alcohol. The Bible warns us, "Wine is a mocker, strong drink is a brawler, and whoever is led astray by it is not wise" (Proverbs 20:1).

Alcohol not only impairs moral judgments, it also impairs our ability to make sensible decisions:

> Tully Isabel Robinson was messaging on her phone, speeding, affected by alcohol, and driving on the wrong side of the road when she crashed into another vehicle, killing its teenage passenger. Robinson, 22, pleaded guilty in the Queenstown District Court on Monday to aggravated careless driving causing the death of Allanah Megan Walker, 17, in a head-on crash on August 22.[42]

There are a million tragic stories just like this, where an innocent life was needlessly taken by someone whose good sense was destroyed by alcohol.

The Bible says, "Do not be drunk with wine, ...but be filled with the Spirit" (Ephesians 5:18). You don't need alcohol to give you boldness. God poured His Spirit out on the Day of Pentecost to give His disciples the boldness to overcome their fear to preach the gospel (see Acts 1:8).

6. Get adequate sleep.

I once wrote a book called *Overcoming Insomnia*[43] in which I share a simple principle for inducing sleep. It is to tire the mind. It's not your body that will keep you awake. It's your overactive mind. Your body may be exhausted, but your thoughts are lining up at a mile a minute as though there's no tomorrow, and you can't stop them. And so you must learn how to still those thoughts.

The Bible tells us how to find rest for our souls. Jesus said,

> "Come to Me, all you who labor and are heavy laden, and I will give you rest. Take My yoke upon you and learn from Me, for I am gentle and lowly in heart, and you will find rest for your souls. For My yoke is easy and My burden is light." (Matthew 11:28–30)

This wonderful promise is often interpreted as "Take all your problems to Jesus and He will fix them." However, the Scriptures tell us to bring our *sins* to Jesus, and He will forgive them. We come to Him laboring and heavy laden with the burden of sin on our back. When He removes it, we find rest for our souls. We no longer have to work to find everlasting life.

7. Wash Your Hands Regularly.

Eating healthy and getting a good night's sleep have a tremendous impact on the strength of our immune system. In addition, there are steps we can take to avoid infection, such as washing our hands frequently and cooking meats thoroughly to prevent food poisoning:

> Carefully wash your hands often, and always before cooking or cleaning. Always wash them again after touching raw meat. Clean dishes and utensils that have had any contact with raw meat, poultry, fish, or eggs.[44]

We take for granted that we are surrounded by an unseen world that can infect our bodies, make us sick, and even kill us if our immune systems are weak. Germs, or what are called "pathogens," are types of microbes that can cause disease. This unseen world wasn't discovered until the advent of the microscope.

The Bible tells us that we live in a world inhabited by unseen spiritual powers:

> For we do not wrestle against flesh and blood, but against principalities, against powers, against the rulers of the darkness of this age, against spiritual hosts of wickedness in the heavenly places. (Ephesians 6:12)

When we sin, we become morally unclean and open ourselves to the diseased demonic world. The Bible says not to "give place to the devil" (Ephesians 4:27). He walks about like a roaring lion, seeking people to devour (1 Peter 5:8). Jesus said that Satan came to kill, steal, and destroy (John 10:10). Serving sin is deadly.

When we are aware of any moral uncleanness, we should therefore immediately confess and forsake it, and we have a promise that God will make us clean:

> If we confess our sins, He is faithful and just to forgive us our sins and to cleanse us from all unrighteousness. (1 John 1:9)

> Who may ascend into the hill of the LORD? Or who may stand in His holy place? He who has clean hands and a pure heart... (Psalm 24:3,4)

8. Manage stress.

Never before in the history of humanity have we had so many conveniences that are designed to make life easier. From flush toilets, hot showers, automatic cars, remote controls, air travel, automatic doors, washing machines, refrigerators, microwaves, and dishwashers, to instant access to information through the Internet, online banking, laptops, iPads, credit cards, smartphones, and even smartwatches that are wearable mini computers. Yet never before have we had so much stress. But there are some practical things the world suggests we can do to help us to manage our stress:

> Modern life is so busy, and sometimes we just need to slow down and chill out. Look at

your life and find small ways you can do that. For example:

- Set your watch 5 to 10 minutes ahead. That way you'll get places a little early and avoid the stress of being late.

- When you're driving on the highway, switch to the slow lane so you can avoid road rage.

- Break down big jobs into smaller ones. For example, don't try to answer all 100 emails if you don't have to—just answer a few of them.[45]

However, the Christian has better ways to manage stress. The world worries about the future, and how they are going to take care of their families and finances. We, instead, simply take the words of Jesus to heart. Most of us are familiar with how He said not to worry about what we eat or drink, and how we should look to the birds in the fields to see how God takes care of them. Here are those marvelous verses:

> "Therefore I say to you, do not worry about your life, what you will eat or what you will drink; nor about your body, what you will put on. Is not life more than food and the body more than clothing? Look at the birds of the air, for they neither sow nor reap nor gather into barns; yet your heavenly Father feeds them. Are you not of more value than

they? Which of you by worrying can add one cubit to his stature?

"So why do you worry about clothing? Consider the lilies of the field, how they grow: they neither toil nor spin; and yet I say to you that even Solomon in all his glory was not arrayed like one of these. Now if God so clothes the grass of the field, which today is, and tomorrow is thrown into the oven, will He not much more clothe you, O you of little faith?

"Therefore do not worry, saying, 'What shall we eat?' or 'What shall we drink?' or 'What shall we wear?' For after all these things the Gentiles seek. For your heavenly Father knows that you need all these things. (Matthew 6:25–32)

However, this passage begins with the word "therefore," and should, therefore, not be read without reading the previous verse. Here is the previous verse:

"No one can serve two masters; for either he will hate the one and love the other, or else he will be loyal to the one and despise the other. You cannot serve God and mammon." (Matthew 6:24)

And there's the key to stress-free living. If we haven't dealt with our love of money, and we are still trusting in it to supply our future needs, we will be plagued with worry. Remember, we *cannot* serve both. It's either God or money. If we love God and we are trusting in Him, we will look to Him alone for our future needs. It is in that trust that we will find peace. This is what is meant by seeking *first* the kingdom of God and His righteousness:

> "But seek first the kingdom of God and His righteousness, and all these things shall be added to you. Therefore do not worry about tomorrow, for tomorrow will worry about its own things. Sufficient for the day is its own trouble." (Matthew 6:33,34)

9. Stay hydrated.

For years I mocked those who daily guzzled large quantities of water, until I developed a very painful kidney stone. When my surgeon said that kidney stones are caused by dehydration, I dove into the daily water-guzzling club.

> Staying adequately hydrated—measured by urine that's light yellow or straw colored—can also help prolong a healthy life by reducing the risk of bladder and colon cancer and keeping kidneys in tip-top shape. Bonus: It might even help you lose weight. Researchers at the University of Illinois found that those who sipped more H_2O ended up eating 68 to 205 fewer calories per day.[46]

Jesus said, "If anyone thirsts, let him come to Me and drink" (John 7:37). Once we understand that everything in this life is temporal and that the Kingdom of God is eternal, we will deliberately order our priorities. Prioritize the cultivation of a disciplined spiritual thirst, and you will keep yourself close to Jesus.

10. Take supplements.

With our diets consisting of highly processed foods, most of us don't get sufficient nutrients from the food we eat. It's good to take supplements to ensure our bodies have all the essential vitamins and minerals we need. Try to find a godly nutritionist who can advise you on what's good and what's not good when it comes to supplements.[47]

There are those who read only the Bible, saying that we don't need supplementary books because they are written by mere men. However, Charles Spurgeon was right when he said, "Give yourself unto reading. The man who never reads will never be read; he who never quotes will never be quoted. He who will not use the thoughts of other men's brains, proves that he has no brains of his own. You need to read."

The Bible says that God Himself gave teachers to the church to feed us spiritually:

> And He Himself gave some to be apostles, some prophets, some evangelists, and some pastors and teachers, for the equipping of the saints for the work of ministry, for the edifying of the body of Christ. (Ephesians 4:11,12)

If we want to grow in our faith, we should read the books of godly teachers, and we should take notice of what they teach.

11. Meditate.

The world suggests meditation, saying that even five minutes a day of simply sitting quietly can make a difference. They say it lowers the heart rate and blood pressure and reduces anxiety.

But again, we have something far better—because we have a worthy object upon which to meditate. We meditate on God and on His Word (see Psalm 1:1–3). Don't just read the Bible as you would a novel. *Meditate* on it. Look for the gold nuggets. Don't be afraid to continually park on one chapter day after day—until you uncover hidden truth:

> This Book of the Law shall not depart from your mouth, but you shall meditate in it day and night, that you may observe to do according to all that is written in it. For then you will make your way prosperous, and then you will have good success. (Joshua 1:8)

12. Get some sun.

Spending some time in natural light is one of the key ways our bodies manufacture vitamin D. Vitamin D plays a role in helping our immune system produce antibodies; low levels of vitamin D, on the other hand, have been correlated with a higher risk of respiratory infection.

Keep yourself in the sunshine of the love of God. Meditate on the sweetness of His love revealed in the cross. That's your source of joy. It's your secret sweet indulgence. In the next chapter we will look closely at an invitation we have to the ultimate feast.

CHAPTER FOURTEEN

YOU'RE INVITED TO DINNER

God's gift of so many delicious foods is in itself an expression of His love for His creation. We have been made with sensitive lips, a tooth-filled mouth, a super-sensitive tongue, thousands of excitable taste buds, and mouth-watering salivary glands. The stomach is a fantastic food factory that hungers to turn the incoming shipment into exported energy.

We also have a *recurring* appetite, without which we would in time wither and die. In the face of all that, we have a smelling nose that is married to our taste buds. Or to put it in a way a child can understand:

When the smell receptors are stimulated, signals travel along the olfactory nerve to the olfactory bulb. The olfactory bulb is underneath the front of your brain just above the nasal cavity. Signals are sent from the olfactory bulb to other parts of the brain to be interpreted as a smell you may recognize, like apple pie fresh from the oven. Yum![48]

We have been fearfully and wonderfully designed by God, not only to eat food, but to eat it with great pleasure. Think of some of those foods, those glorious foods—besides that freshly baked apple pie and ice cream, there is the sight and smell of golden fried chicken and mashed potatoes dripping with gravy, the first bite of a salty potato chip, explosively delicious French fries, a tender T-bone steak, fresh bread dripping with melted butter, crispy bacon, and of course that deliriously delicious and decadent indulgence—chocolate. Think of juicy pears, bunches of sweet grapes, bright red strawberries, carefully arranged orange oranges, colorful watermelons, bright yellow lemons, crispy apple strudels, and schnitzel with noodles—these are a few of my favorite things.

How kind God is to make such amazing fruits, each of which is kept in good supply because every one of them contains tiny miraculous seeds—giving them the ability to reproduce themselves. And we don't have to be rich to enjoy these natural pleasures. They are within easy reach of all of us when we trust "in the living God, *who gives us richly all things to enjoy* (1 Timothy 6:17).

When Paul and Barnabas spoke to their hearers at Lystra, they said,

"Nevertheless He did not leave Himself without witness, in that He did good, gave us rain from heaven and fruitful seasons, *filling our hearts with food and gladness.*" (Acts 14:17)

Look at how the disciples relished a good meal:

So continuing daily with one accord in the temple, and breaking bread from house to house, they ate their food with gladness and simplicity of heart… (Acts 2:46)

And one thing we can do is share that eating experience with others. This is what Jesus often did. He chose His company carefully, and in Luke chapter 15, He used food as a plate to serve up a threefold sermon, which in itself, culminated in a celebratory feast.

He gave his hearers two parables, both illustrating the value of something that had been lost. One was just a common sheep, and the other was an inanimate object—a mere coin. But then He elevated the lost-and-found principle with a third story, one of a lost human being—a special creation that had been made in the image of God:

Then He said: "A certain man had two sons. And the younger of them said to his father, 'Father, give me the portion of goods that falls to me.' So he divided to them his livelihood. And not many days after, the younger son gathered all together, journeyed to a far country, and there wasted his possessions with prodigal living." (Luke 15:11–13)

Not many days after, the son "gathered all together." He couldn't wait to gather his possessions—everything he had—and leave. His gathering of all of his possessions shows that he didn't plan on coming back. His hormones had kicked in, and later on in the story we find that he wanted to visit prostitutes. Perhaps he had expressed his desires to his older brother, because his brother knew why he left. Maybe the prodigal had asked his brother to join him to indulge in sexual pleasure. Whatever the case, upon the prodigal's return, the elder brother spilled the beans:

> "But as soon as this son of yours came, who has devoured your livelihood with harlots…" (Luke 15:30)

That's why the son journeyed to a *far* country! He wanted to get away from his father—because he knew that he would frown upon his sexual aspirations. Perhaps his father had him memorize some relevant Scripture:

> For why should you, my son, be enraptured by an immoral woman, and be embraced in the arms of a seductress? For the ways of man are before the eyes of the Lord, and He ponders all his paths. His own iniquities entrap the wicked man, and he is caught in the cords of his sin. (Proverbs 5:20–22)

He *had* to get away from his father, and get as far away as possible. And in that desire we see traces of Adam—still running and hiding from God because of his sin.

As the story unfolds, the prodigal begins to be in want:

> "But when he had spent all, there arose a severe famine in that land, and he began to be in want. Then he went and joined himself to a citizen of that country, and he sent him into his fields to feed swine. And he would gladly have filled his stomach with the pods that the swine ate, and no one gave him anything.
>
> "But when he came to himself, he said, 'How many of my father's hired servants have bread enough and to spare, and I perish with hunger!'" (Luke 15:14–17)

The gnawing of his hunger pangs reminded him of the providence of his benevolent father. His hired servants had bread enough to spare, while he was dying of starvation. Hidden here is a most precious gem. He wasn't just hungering for his father's food. He was so hungry that he was desiring the filthy food the pigs were eating. It was that sobering revelation that brought him to his senses.

And that's the revelation that will bring us to our senses. We are made in the glorious image of Almighty God. We're not thoughtless beasts. And yet our consuming desire is for that which is unclean. We rummage around in the filth of sin—driven by an incessant sexual appetite—our eyes are *full* of adultery. And all this God sees: "For the ways of man are before the eyes of the LORD, and He ponders all his paths" (Proverbs 5:21).

This starving prodigal suddenly had serious thoughts of God. Look at what he said, and what then happened:

> " 'I will arise and go to my father, and will say to him, "Father, I have sinned against heaven and before you, and I am no longer worthy to be called your son. Make me like one of your hired servants." '
>
> "And he arose and came to his father. But when he was still a great way off, his father saw him and had compassion, and ran and fell on his neck and kissed him. And the son said to him, 'Father, I have sinned against heaven and in your sight, and am no longer worthy to be called your son.'
>
> "But the father said to his servants, 'Bring out the best robe and put it on him, and put a ring on his hand and sandals on his feet. And bring the fatted calf here and kill it, and let us eat and be merry; for this my son was dead and is alive again; he was lost and is found.' And they began to be merry." (Luke 15:18–24)

That's a picture of God watching for the lost sinner, rejoicing in our repentance, celebrating that we were once dead in our trespasses and that we are now alive in Christ.

God has saved us from death, and we will one day gloriously celebrate all this at what Scripture calls "the marriage supper of the Lamb." That feast will make the most breathtaking and mouthwatering table spread look like the dregs at the bottom of a dumpster:

> "Let us be glad and rejoice and give Him glory, for the marriage of the Lamb has come, and His wife has made herself ready." And to her it was granted to be arrayed in fine linen, clean and bright, for the fine linen is the righteous acts of the saints.
>
> Then he said to me, "Write: 'Blessed are those who are called to the marriage supper of the Lamb!'" (Revelation 19:7–9)

And now, those who are servants of Christ have been commanded by Jesus to invite others:

> "The kingdom of heaven is like a certain king who arranged a marriage for his son, and sent out his servants to call those who were invited to the wedding; and they were not willing to come. Again, he sent out other servants, saying, 'Tell those who are invited, "See, I have prepared my dinner; my oxen and fatted cattle are killed, and all things are ready. Come to the wedding."'…
>
> "Then he said to his servants, 'The wedding is ready, but those who were invited

> were not worthy. Therefore go into the high-
> ways, and as many as you find, invite to the
> wedding.' So those servants went out into the
> highways and gathered together all whom
> they found, both bad and good. And the
> wedding hall was filled with guests." (Mat-
> thew 22:2–4,8–10)

The good and bad were gathered together. Keep
in mind that the church is made up of true and false
converts who have been gathered together. The
sheep and goats will be alongside each other until
they are sorted out on the Day of Judgment (see
Matthew 25:31–33):

> "But when the king came in to see the guests,
> he saw a man there who did not have on a
> wedding garment. So he said to him, 'Friend,
> how did you come in here without a wedding
> garment?' And he was speechless. Then the
> king said to the servants, 'Bind him hand and
> foot, take him away, and cast him into outer
> darkness; there will be weeping and gnashing
> of teeth.'
>   "For many are called, but few are cho-
> sen." (Matthew 22:11–14)

Think of this frightening scene. This was a wedding guest who thought that he was there legiti-
mately. But he wasn't. He wasn't wearing a wedding
garment. This is a picture of many who have named
the name of Christ, but have never departed from
their sin. In other words, they thought they were

Christians, but they were living lives of hypocrisy. They were self-deceived. To be cast out of an expected Heaven into the horror of Hell would be the ultimate nightmare. I hope that's not a picture of you. I hope that you have genuinely repented—that you're trusting in Jesus alone, and that you're no longer serving sin.

One evidence that you *are* genuinely saved is that you will have a deep-rooted love for God and a love for your fellow human beings. That means you will care about the unsaved, and you will want to reach them with the gospel.

Consider this story that Jesus told about a rich man who dined lavishly *every* day:

> "There was a certain rich man who was clothed in purple and fine linen and fared sumptuously every day. But there was a certain beggar named Lazarus, full of sores, who was laid at his gate, desiring to be fed with the crumbs which fell from the rich man's table. Moreover the dogs came and licked his sores." (Luke 16:19–21)

The rich man had no love for the poor man at his gate. He let him starve while he fed his selfish face. Then Jesus explained what happened after they both died:

> "So it was that the beggar died, and was carried by the angels to Abraham's bosom. The rich man also died and was buried. And

being in torments in Hades [Hell], he lifted up his eyes and saw Abraham afar off, and Lazarus in his bosom.

"Then he cried and said, 'Father Abraham, have mercy on me, and send Lazarus that he may dip the tip of his finger in water and cool my tongue; for I am tormented in this flame.' But Abraham said, 'Son, remember that in your lifetime you received your good things, and likewise Lazarus evil things; but now he is comforted and you are tormented. And besides all this, between us and you there is a great gulf fixed, so that those who want to pass from here to you cannot, nor can those from there pass to us.'" (Luke 16:22–26)

These words of Scripture fly in the face of those who maintain that "Hell" is just a word the Bible uses for the grave, or that it's merely a reference to a burning trash heap outside of Jerusalem. Listen to the rich man's desperate plea to Abraham:

"Then he said, 'I beg you therefore, father, that you would send him to my father's house, for I have five brothers, that he may testify to them, lest they also come to this place of torment.' Abraham said to him, 'They have Moses and the prophets; let them hear them.' And he said, 'No, father Abraham; but if one goes to them from the dead, they will repent.' But he said to him, 'If they do not hear Moses and the prophets, neither will they be persuaded though one rise from the dead.'" (Luke 16:27–31)

This is more than a story about a man who liked to eat but didn't care about the poor. We know from Scripture that we don't enter Heaven because we feed needy people. We are saved by God's grace alone without works (see Ephesians 2:8,9).

Perhaps this is a story of the rich and self-indulgent church—the church that has no concern that sinners are starving at their gate for want of the Bread of Life. These who profess faith in Jesus are interested in everything but the task of reaching the lost. I hope that's not you. I hope that you desperately want to see people come to a knowledge of salvation.

Eternal Salivation

If you don't know the Lord, right now, come to your senses. I wrote this book for *you*—because I want to see you in Heaven. I shudder at the thought of you going to Hell. Please, get up and leave the pigsty of sin. Put your trust in Jesus. Let Him clothe you with a robe of righteousness. This promise is for you:

"Blessed are those who hunger and thirst for righteousness, for they shall be filled." (Matthew 5:6)

So is this one:

Why do you spend money for what is not bread, and your wages for what does not satisfy? Listen carefully to Me, and eat what is good, and let your soul delight itself in abundance. Incline your ear, and come to Me. Hear, and your soul shall live... (Isaiah 55:2,3)

God Himself is running to you as the father did to his beloved prodigal son. He is inviting you to the marriage supper of the Lamb. Your presence is requested. Will you come? RSVP. Whatever you do, don't make light of it. Don't put it off until tomorrow. To put it off *is* to make light of it. *Today* if you hear His voice, don't harden your heart:

And the Spirit and the bride say, "Come!" And let him who hears say, "Come!" And let him who thirsts come. Whoever desires, let him take the water of life freely. (Revelation 22:17)

We are waiting for a new heavens and a new earth. There is no food, no feast, no beautiful flower, no breathtaking sunrise or sunset, nor delirious pleasure that anywhere near compares to that which God has prepared for those who love Him:

But as it is written:

"Eye has not seen, nor ear heard,
Nor have entered into the heart of man
The things which God has prepared for
those who love Him." (1 Corinthians 2:9)

Don't be like the man Jesus said was a fool—because he stored all his riches on earth and ignored Heaven.

In Your presence is fullness of joy; at Your right hand are pleasures forevermore. (Psalm 16:11)

NOTES

1. naturenates.com/does-honey-expire/
2. kingjamesbibledictionary.com/Dictionary/honey
3. "6 Dangerous Side Effects of Eating Too Much Butter, According to Experts"; eatthis.com/news-side-effects-eating-too-much-butter/
4. scientificamerican.com/article/is-butter-a-healthy-fat/
5. "Is Butter Really Back? | Harvard Public Health Magazine | Harvard T.H. Chan School of Public Health" hsph.harvard.edu/magazine/magazine_article/is-butter-really-back/
6. "4 Ways Margarine is Bad For Your Heart"; culinary nutrition.com/4-ways-margarine-is-bad-for-your-heart/
7. "Butter vs. Margarine - Harvard Health"; health.harvard.edu/staying-healthy/butter-vs-margarine
8. healthline.com/nutrition/15-health-foods-that-are-really-junk-foods
9. westonaprice.org/health-topics/know-your-fats/why-butter-is-better/
10. kids.britannica.com/students/article/butter/273419
11. "Did Jesus Eat Fish?" | PETA; petalambs.com/features/jesus-eat-fish/
12. "Why did Jesus Eat Fish? – Swords to Plowshares"; swords2plowshares.com/2018/05/13/why-did-jesus-eat-fish/
13. blueletterbible.org/lexicon/g3795/kjv/tr/0-1/
14. en.wikipedia.org/wiki/Ancient_Israelite_cuisine

15. news.discovery.com/history/religion/last-supper-menu-stew-lamb-wine-of-course-more150402.htm
16. lifeway.com/en/articles/biblical-illustrator-preparing-for-passover
17. allmychefs.com/ingredients/veal_858
18. 21gourmetstreet.com/gourmet-talk/healthy-food-veal-low-calorie/
19. "Salt: The Silent Killer," John D, Day, MD, April 5, 2013; intermountainhealthcare.org/blogs/topics/heart/2013/04/salt-the-silent-killer/
20. "Controversy Over Salt Restrictions"; hmpgloballearning network.com/site/pln/blog/controversy-over-salt-restrictions
21. Science News: "Pass the salt: Study finds average consumption safe for heart health"; sciencedaily.com/releases/2018/08/180809202057.htm
22. webmd.com/a-to-z-guides/why-are-tears-salty
23. en.wikipedia.org/wiki/Ancient_Israelite_cuisine
24. "Are Eggs Good For You? | Eggs and Cholesterol"; runnersworld.com/news/a26868477/are-eggs-healthy/
25. Ibid.
26. biblestudytools.com/commentaries/gills-exposition-of-the-bible/psalms-104-15.html
27. "How Our Bodies Turn Food Into Energy"; healthy.kaiser permanente.org/washington/health-wellness/healtharticle. how-our-bodies-turn-food-into-energy
28. en.wikipedia.org/wiki/Ancient_Israelite_cuisine
29. cbsnews.com/news/cristiano-ronaldo-coca-cola-market-value-loss/
30. ligonier.org/learn/articles/cursing-fig-tree/
31. thegospelcoalition.org/article/jesus-curse-fig-tree/
32. biblehub.com/commentaries/matthew/21-19.htm
33. en.wikipedia.org/wiki/Ancient_Israelite_cuisine
34. Transcription from YouTube (Living Waters): "Food: The Key to Long Life" (9:10–28:50); youtu.be/_FxMk8zXkf8
35. gotquestions.org/this-is-my-body-broken-for-you.html
36. "Why you should steam your veggies"; sciencenorway.no/a/1430207
37. foodforlife.com/about_us/ezekiel-49

38. tcho.com/blogs/news/8-potential-health-benefits-of-the-theobromine-found-in-chocolate; healthline.com/nutrition/7-health-benefits-dark-chocolate

39. allthatsinteresting.com/jeanne-calment

40. Tilapia is probably the oldest farm raised fish in the world. Stories from biblical scholars suggest it was the fish used by Jesus to feed the crowds at the Sea of Galilee…Today, over 80 nations produce farm-raised tilapia including the United States. China is the largest producer accounting for over 50 percent of the world's production. www.seafoodhealthfacts.org/description-top-commercial-seafood-items/tilapia

41. healthline.com/health/alcohol/effects-on-body

42. stuff.co.nz/national/crime/125506101/driver-messaging-on-facebook-at-time-of-crash-that-killed-teenager

43. A reader posted the following review on our website: "Recently you offered *Overcoming Insomnia* as a weekend special for $1 per book. I was skeptical that you would be able to deliver a book that would be medically informative to sleep disorder patients. I only ordered 50 (I wish I had ordered 200 more), I have never read a better book for patients that covers the basics of sleep disorders. Since we are an independent sleep lab I am able to give every patient one of your books. Thank you for doing such excellent work." — Tony Huff, RPSGT, RST, Georgetown Sleep, KY.

44. "Preventing food poisoning"; medlineplus.gov/ency/article/007441.htm

45. webmd.com/balance/guide/tips-to-control-stress

46. aarp.org/health/healthy-living/info-2017/50-ways-to-live-longer.html

47. My personal nutritionist is Dr. James Augustine; aheadto wellness.com/dr-james-augustine/

48. kidshealth.org/en/kids/nose.html

RESOURCES

If you have not yet placed your trust in Jesus Christ and would like additional information, please check out the following helpful resources:

How to Know God Exists. Clear evidences for His existence will convince you that belief in God is reasonable and rational—a matter of fact and not faith.

The Evidence Study Bible. Answers to over 200 questions, thousands of comments, and 130 informative articles will help you better comprehend the Christian faith.

Why Christianity? (DVD). If you have ever asked what happens after we die, if there is a Heaven, or how good we have to be to go there, this DVD will help you.

See our YouTube channel (youtube.com/livingwaters) to watch free movies such as "The Atheist Delusion," "Evolution vs. God," "Crazy Bible," as well as thousands of other fascinating videos.

If you are a new believer, please read *Save Yourself Some Pain*, written just for you (available free online at LivingWaters.com, or as a booklet).

For more resources, visit LivingWaters.com, call 800-437-1893, or write to: Living Waters Publications, P.O. Box 1172, Bellflower, CA 90707.